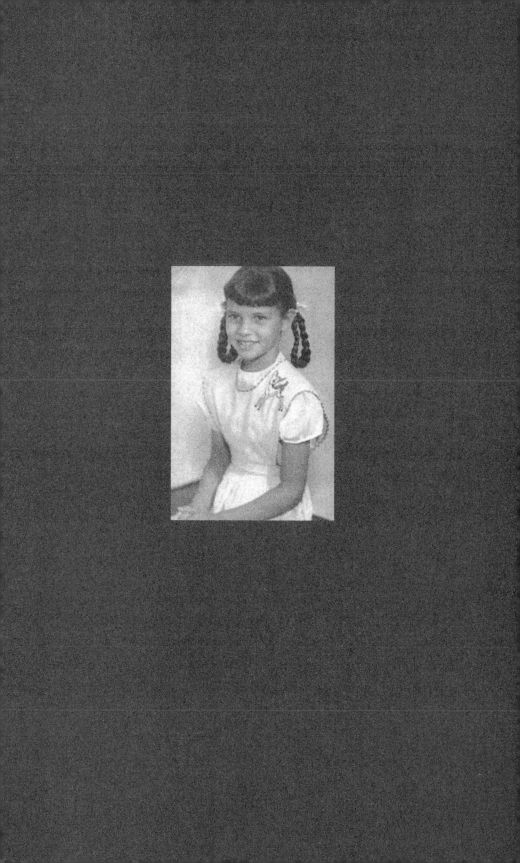

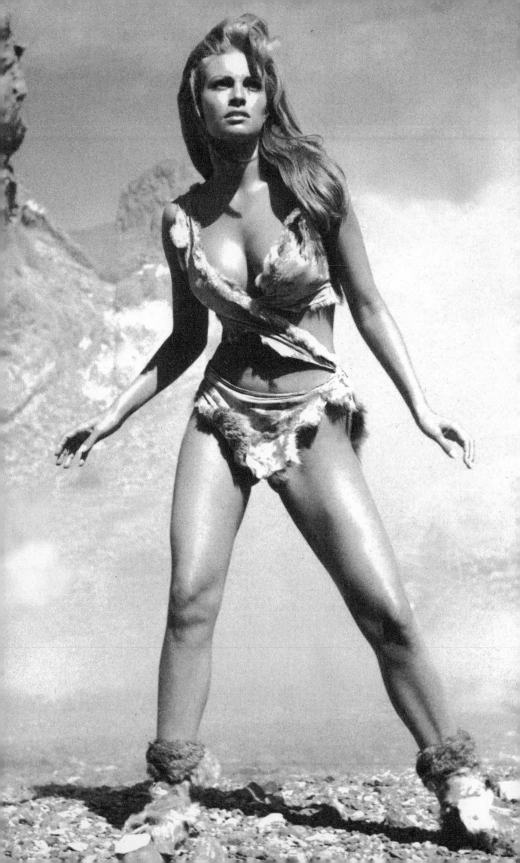

RAQUEL WELCH

Beyond the Cleavage

WEINSTEIN
BOOKS

Credits beginning on page 273 constitute a continuation of the copyright page.

ISBN: 978-1-60286-097-1

First Edition
10 9 8 7 6 5 4 3 2 1

For Damon and Tahnee
with all my love

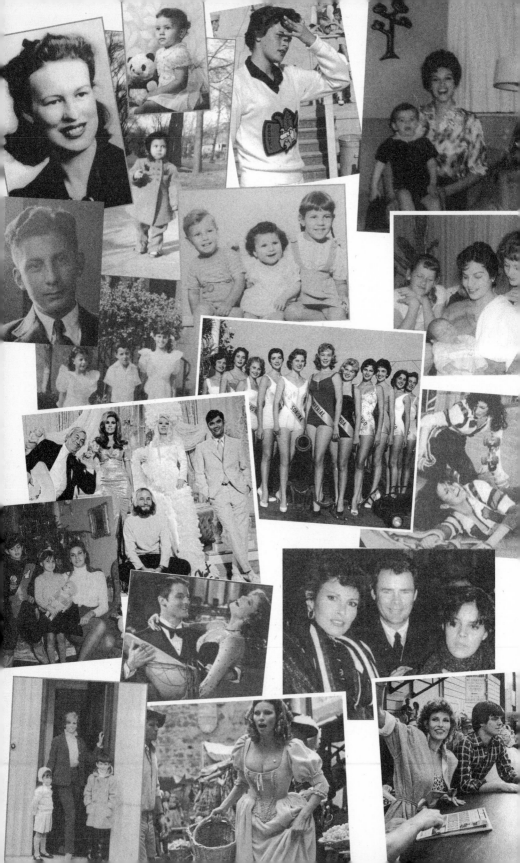

CONTENTS

Preface

THOUGH YOU MAY KNOW WHO I AM AND
what I look like after all these years, it's safe to say that you don't really
know much about me. How could you? I'm usually a very private person and allow people to make whatever assumptions they will from my
public image in various films and television appearances.

So before I start spouting off, it's only fair to bring you a little
closer into my confidence and let you know something about myself. In
a sense I'm using the occasion of this book to say a lot of things I've
never said before. It's a change for me to air my opinions publicly and
to share what kind of person I've become . . . now that I've grown older.
Indeed, through most of my professional life I've been seen and not
heard. So now that the passing years have given me plenty to say and
the courage to say it, I hope you can find something in my words that
serves you.

This is a book not only about aging, but also about coming of age.
For me, getting older has been about coming into my own and finally
getting to the point where I'm not afraid to speak my mind. We are,
without question, living in a very turbulent and pivotal time in history.
I don't recognize my country anymore, or the role of women in this
world of vanishing moral values. Our culture seems to be in the throes
of change, but who knows what will emerge in its place. I am cheered
by the knowledge that we women have broken through the proverbial
glass ceiling, rising to the forefront of the political scene, both as vice-
presidential and presidential candidates. More and more we are part of
contemporary social commentary and can, I hope, provide a steady
compass for the future. I am further emboldened throughout the pages
of this book to speak candidly about the lost art of being a woman; about
aging, lifestyles, love, sex, forgiveness, and . . . Well, read on and you'll
get to know me better.

RAQUEL

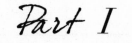

Part I

BEING
A
WOMAN

ONE

Behind the Myth

CONTRARY TO POPULAR MYTH, I DIDN'T JUST hatch out of an eagle's nest, circa *One Million Years B.C.*, clad in a doe-skin bikini. In fact, I was more surprised than anyone to find myself on location in such an exotic setting, high atop a volcanic mountain in the Canary Islands! With the release of that famous movie poster, in one fell swoop, everything in my life changed and everything about the real me was swept away. All else would be eclipsed by this bigger-than-life sex symbol.

She came into public consciousness as a physical presence, without a voice. How could I hope to survive such an unpredictable beginning, and learn to carry the baggage that came with it? *One Million Years B.C.* was only my second film for 20th Century Fox. I had no other credentials as an actress outside of that one laughable line of dialogue: "Me Loana . . . You Tumak." It felt like I'd stumbled into a booby trap— pun intended. I am living proof that a picture speaks a thousand words. It seems like everything that's happened to me since has flowed from that moment, frozen in time.

The irony of it all is that even though people thought of me as a sex symbol, in reality I was a single mother of two small children! It's true! However, nobody would have believed it back then, not when they saw me in that skimpy fur bikini. Can you picture the girl in the poster with a baby in one arm and pushing a stroller with the other? Kind of destroys the fantasy, doesn't it? Ironically, I am duty bound and destined to do just that.

My task of destroying the myth is long overdue. It's an absolute necessity to pull back the veil, so to speak, in order to make way for the authentic *me*. So let's flash back in time to almost seventy years ago and retrace the steps of my real life.

World War II

I was born in 1940 in the Windy City, Chicago. Not ideal for a newborn baby girl with thin Mediterranean blood, courtesy of my Spanish father. For my first outing, I was bundled into a snowsuit to protect me from the very, very cold weather. Luckily for me, my folks moved to California when I was barely two; a good thing, because my baby brain was frozen solid until that point. That's probably why I've had an aversion to anything cold ever since, from icy drinks to frigid people.

Happy in the warm glow of the California sunshine, my baby brain thawed and I became a much more smiley toddler in the Golden State of Boredom. My father worked as an aeronautical engineer in San Diego, designing aircraft at General Dynamics. It was wartime, so we lived in government housing, called "the projects" in the Mission Bay area. The units were almost like military barracks. Up until I was five, I would save the tinfoil from my gum wrappers for the war effort. Everybody pitched in back then.

My mother was Anglo. Her ancestry dated back to John Quincy Adams and the *Mayflower*. My father was born into a good family in La Paz, Bolivia. I was the first of their three children. My father had been hoping for a firstborn son and got me instead. He didn't have much regard for the female of the species, unless they were parading around in swimsuits. Do you get the picture? My brother, James Stanford — called Jim — was hatched on exactly the same day as me, two years later, on September 5. My younger sister, Gayle Carole, came along one year later.

Even though Mom, Dad, and two-year-old me ended up in Southern California where the sun outside was always shining, it was strangely chilly inside our family home. Physical affection was in short supply. There was no cuddling or lovey-dovey stuff happening, even between Mom and Dad. I don't recall ever seeing him kiss her or hold her hand. I was left hungry for a taste of tenderness and romance from an early age. All of us were terrified of my father. He was quick to anger and was a stickler for manners and rules in our modest home. I complied.

As a kid, I had a highly emotional nature and loved being swept away on flights of imagination. Inside my head, anything could happen, and I could avoid the fact that I felt trapped under the thumb of my domineering father. In my mind, I was already grown-up and independent. I was simply waiting for the biological process to catch up with my vision . . . so I could escape. I had to wait to reclaim my childhood until after I left home.

I grew up with one ear glued to the radio. Our family gathered 'round it to hear Roosevelt's speeches, and I also knew all the words to the popular tunes on the airwaves. I would sing them around the house, in the car, and on the backyard swing. My favorites were *Don't Fence Me In* and *I'm Looking over a Four Leaf Clover.* My father used to call me out to the living room to sing for company. It was kind of embarrassing, but I did it anyway. I got the early impression that above all else, I was on this planet to make my moody dad proud of me.

Later on, we got a brand-new television set, complete with rabbit ears and fuzzy black-and-white reception. There were lots of comedy shows, with Jackie Gleason, Red Skelton, Milton Berle, and Sid Caesar; but my fave was Jerry Lewis. I used to squeal with laughter over his childish antics. He seemed like a big overgrown kid. By the time I grew up, I had switched my attention to Dean Martin, the suave, handsome crooner. Years later, I would actually get the chance to star in a movie with Dean and Jimmy Stewart!

What's in a Name?

Just as the war ended, in 1945, so did my kindergarten class. A dark cloud had been lifted, and we moved out of "the projects" and across the bay into a real house, with roses growing over a trellis; a yard filled with peach, plum, and avocado trees; and a dog named Shep. Dad drove a Hudson. It was the American dream! It was also a new neighborhood, and I changed schools just in time to enter first grade at Bay Park Grammar School.

I was registered with my full name: Jo-Raquel Tejada. Quite a mouthful. No one could pronounce it. My schoolmates started calling me "Jo." No matter how many times I tried to tell them, "I'm not Jo. I'm Raquel," I couldn't make them stop. One day, my mother showed up at the administration office and scratched the "Jo" off the school record. Gone were those two letters that bound me to her, since I'd been named after her—Jo was short for Josephine. The only problem in deleting it was that "Jo" was the only part of my name that anyone could *pronounce*. Why couldn't I be a Mary Smith? I didn't like being so different. But I was, and in time, I would learn to embrace my "Raquelness."

I had no idea how I got the name Raquel Tejada. I had just accepted it. But now the question had been raised and was begging for an answer. It turns out that I'd been named after my paternal grandmother, Raquel, whom I had never even seen. She lived in La Paz, and I didn't meet her until I was thirty-two. The name "Tejada," Mom explained, came from the name for the type of spear carried by the king's royal guards in sixteenth-century Spain. I couldn't relate.

Dad seemed indifferent to his heritage and never spoke of his childhood, his siblings or parents, or anything personal. For most of my life, he was an enigma to me. He spoke only occasionally of his Bolivian roots, and he never spoke Spanish in our home. This made me feel like there was something wrong with being from Bolivia, "a third-world country." It was troubling, but I didn't ask about it. I was only six years old and didn't want to know the answer. For now, if the kids at school could just get my name right, I'd settle for that. By the time I hit high school, everyone called me Rocky.

Over time, I came to think that my father's willful disconnect must have made him feel very lonely and isolated at times, which would account for his moods. This presented me with some serious issues to work through. Was my dad ashamed of his Latin heritage? I chose not to think so, to sidestep feeling ashamed myself. On a childish, subliminal level, I actually did understand why he was not forthcoming about his background. It was because he had divorced his family and his country to come to the fabled U.S.A., the land of opportunity. There was no going back. He had made a commitment, and it was clear that he was now, first and foremost, an American.

Mom, on the other hand, had a drawer in which she kept photographs of the two years she'd spent in La Paz with my father, after they were first married and before I was born. We went through all her souvenir pictures of Bolivia together. There were shots of the Indians in derby hats and long braids and the exotic boats they crafted for sailing on the fabled Lake Titicaca. There were also pictures of Dad posing in a fedora, showing how desolate the terrain was on the Alto Plano high above the city of La Paz. I always wondered why all this memorabilia was kept hidden in the bottom of a drawer.

Despite everything that remained unspoken, I did learn that Dad was one of six children. I would be sixty years old before I set foot in my father's birthplace of La Paz. When I was growing up it seemed like a very far off planet.

Mom vs. Dad

My mother, Josephine Sarah Hall, was a real lady. She had a beautiful smile, which she wore easily and often; and though she was soft-spoken, she was a dynamo. I came to realize that she was anything but weak. She had enormous inner resources and a powerful will. Despite this, my father had the upper hand.

Mom was a great seamstress. She made all our clothes on her Singer sewing machine. I cannot imagine whipping up some of the things she did. It's like an ancient skill from another century. Gayle and I always had the same Easter dresses, but in different colors. (See the photo of Gayle, Jim, and me in the photo insert.) I was very proud of my dresses and have always admired women who could make clothes from scratch. I am missing that gene.

My mother also had a job. She used to get up at the crack of dawn to get ready for work, and I would sit on the edge of the tub and watch her apply makeup in the bathroom mirror. She gave me all my ideas about how a woman should be. She never wore rollers or pin curls around the house, and neither would I. Her wardrobe was always co-ordinated, and she was smart and articulate. She was a college gradu-ate from the University of Illinois, where she had met my father. She was a hardworking person who put forth a tremendous amount of ef-fort toward cooking, cleaning, laundry, yard work (cutting the hedges and mowing the lawn) *and* washing our cars. Oh, and she also did the ironing and the baking and chauffeured us kids from here to there. She was really something!

Mom used to read wonderful Hans Christian Andersen fairy tales to us at bedtime. It would be a special treat when she'd linger to scratch my back before tucking me in. She was also a churchgoer who enrolled us all in Daily Vacation Bible School every summer. I went every year until I was thirteen. We weren't particularly religious per se, but Mom attended church every Sunday with all three of us kids in tow . . . dressed up and polished. We attended the Pacific Beach Presbyterian Church. Dad only went on Easter and Christmas.

One thing about church was that people were dressed nicely and on their best behavior. This was, of course, a bit boring for a fidgety child, but it gave me a sense of what decency looked like. My mother, as well, was a perfect example of that.

When it came to my father, everyone walked on eggshells. We all avoided him for fear of criticism or a cruel remark about our appear-ance. We had to watch what we said, what we wore, how we combed our hair . . . everything came under his scrutiny, especially our grades in school. Sometimes he'd demand that I sit next to him on the couch and read aloud from *Time* magazine or *Newsweek* without any mistakes. It was hit or miss; he could be quite reasonable, even charming . . . but you never knew when he'd "fly off the handle," as Mom used to put it.

When that happened, we would run to Mother. There was no place else to go. She might try, but she was no match for him. Jo, as *she* liked to be called, was far too timid around my father. Even as a child I was acutely aware of this dynamic between the two and didn't like it one bit. I could tell that Mom was scared of Dad, which made me feel terribly vulnerable. Who would protect us? Eventually, that someone turned out to be me.

We all had our escape routes planned. Most of the time, whoever "got it" first was cooked, because the other two kids would run for cover, leaving the first victim to bear the brunt of my father's anger. Usually, that was my brother Jim. Dad always went for him first. I guess because he was the boy. That made Gayle and me feel horribly guilty. Boy, was I glad that I didn't have to bear the burden of being a son.

Facing the Dragon

Every time Dad lashed out at my mother, *I* flinched—it might as well have been me! I felt the need to vindicate her, but was helpless to do so. I crossed that bridge when I finally confronted my dad in defense of my mother, and this time he *had* to back down. I'll never forget that moment as long as I live. I was sixteen . . . and had had enough. We had just sat down for dinner when Dad began complaining about the casserole Mom had served. Suddenly, he picked up his glass of milk from the table and threw it right in her face. It was the worst thing I could ever imagine, seeing her look of shock, watching her sit there with her face and hair drenched and dripping, humiliated. I couldn't believe my eyes. All this over something he didn't like about the meal? My poor mother was reduced to a whimpering mess . . . defeated.

That was it. Tears streaming, I jumped up from the table and went for the fireplace, as he came after me. "Where do you think you're going?" he demanded.

"How could you?" I screamed, and picked up the poker from the fireplace and turned toward him, gripping it with both hands. I was pitted against him now. "If you ever, ever do anything to hurt Mom again, I swear, I'll kill you!" I said, shaking with emotion. He glared at me and stood his ground. "Calm down," he said. I glared right back at him.

Thank God, he backed away. I cannot believe I am telling this about someone I loved so much. Everything I did was to please him. But someone had to stand up to him. And as the oldest, that someone was me.

I remember vividly the adrenaline rush I got from walking up to the dragon and discovering that I was no longer afraid. That moment also included an epiphany about my father. I sensed his vulnerability. I could see in him the young man of seventeen who had come to this country from Bolivia with dreams of science, space, and aeronautics. I could see the man who had learned to speak impeccable English and studied engineering at the university where he met my mother. He had lifted himself up, lifting me up with him. I saw how his internal struggle, his drive and his masculine pride had been tested to the limit, sometimes to the breaking point, which accounted for his lousy temper. I didn't excuse him . . . but I suddenly understood him. This helped later when it was time for me to forgive.

Not under His Thumb

My mother was under my father's thumb. I sure didn't want to be like her in that respect. But I think I am like her in other ways. Anyway, I got the feminine part down pat. But when it came to deferring to a male who was demanding? Not so much. That's where my mom and I differ radically. By observing my mother in her relationship with my father, I learned that women have different roles to play. I think she was right about that part. However, after four husbands, I don't think I'm a good candidate for wifedom. I like my independence too much.

A life of female servitude doesn't appeal to me mainly because I saw my mother being taken for granted. I don't have memories of any appreciation coming her way. Between my parents there was not the slightest gesture of fondness; no hand-holding or sitting close with arms around each other; and hardly ever a kiss. As the song goes, "Try a little tenderness." Where, oh where, was that tenderness? I wondered. Where was his appreciation for all she did as a wife, mother, and homemaker? Men who behave like that have only themselves to blame for the backlash.

My romantic life would be something quite different. I wasn't ever willing to settle for the dry, estranged relationship of my parents. I'm allergic to it. I knew I couldn't (and wouldn't) tolerate it. I suppose that in some way, I wanted to vindicate my mother's suffering and selflessness. Oh boy . . . Who can control the subconscious mind? Where was mine leading me?

When I put myself in my mother's shoes, I thought how I would have walked out on my father long ago. It used to frustrate me that she put up with it. When I was about sixteen, I asked her why she'd stayed and didn't leave. She said it was for us, the children. She wanted us to finish school before she would even consider such a thing.

Escaping Reality

I was at the mercy of my turbulent family life. Like many children, my imagination allowed me to slip from the bounds of my dysfunctional family and invent another world to inhabit. Make-believe was a lovely place to be, and I could control it. It seemed as if I had always wanted to be an actress. Mom was encouraging, but no one pushed me into it. I took it upon *myself* to stir up some action, Andy Hardy–style, and started to put on plays in our garage using blue chenille bedspreads for curtains. All the neighbors came, and the kids on our block played the various parts.

Mercifully, my mother soon realized I was a budding performer and enrolled me in the San Diego Junior Theatre, an annex of San Diego's Old Globe. In my first play, I was surprised to be cast as the prince in *The Princess and the Caterpillar*. A boy! Why a boy? I was only seven, but it bothered me. Wasn't I pretty enough to be the princess?

Meanwhile, the more I performed, the more my father smiled and tapped his knee, in a kind of excited fashion. It was a good sign. But I had to be careful about that tapping. It might turn into a ticking time bomb.

At about the same time, Daddy took me to see the movie *The Red Shoes*. As I watched Moira Shearer dance herself into feverish abandon in the film, she quickly became my new idol. I was under the spell of her magical red toe shoes. It pitched my romantic temperament into high gear, and that was when I began to take ballet lessons. Ballet would become a consuming passion—especially in my teenage years—and a lasting influence in my life. I started classical ballet at age seven and continued to study dance for the next ten years, and even after I graduated from high school.

Not surprisingly, I developed a schoolgirl crush on my ballet teacher, Irene Isham Clark. She cut quite a striking figure with her long silver hair cascading down her back, well past her waist. She would put it up with exotic-looking combs during class. Irene Clark was not at all like the typical La Jolla matron. She was an *artiste*. She conducted class by tapping an ornately carved cane with a silver tip like a rhythmic metronome to the count of *Les Sylphides*.

Then came the day when this ballet goddess broke my heart. When I was seventeen, Irene told me that I would never become a classical ballerina. She thought I would make a better comedienne. Although I was crushed, she turned out to be right, and I just had to live with it. But all those years of devotion to dance didn't go to waste. By my midteens, the ballet classes had shaped a near-perfect body.

Puberty

By age thirteen a truckload of hormonal changes had come raining down on me. I was emotionally still a girl, but now suddenly I was becoming a young woman. It was frightening. Nature was running its course and pubescent girls had to just sit helplessly waiting, during what amounted to a high-stakes poker game, nervously watching to see what cards they would be dealt in the game of life.

Dad said I had racehorse legs. Was that a good thing? Anyway, I was broad shouldered, small waisted, and slim hipped with new rosebud boobies starting to blossom. What should I do about it? It was embarrassing and reassuring at the same time. It seemed too early to start becoming . . . a woman. Then, suddenly and mysteriously, lovely things began happening to me. Nature was working its magic, transforming Raquel Tejada into someone else.

However, the game was playing out slowly, taking its time over a period of a couple of years. Whereas for some girls it was one summer — and *whamo!* — girl to woman at the speed of light, for me it was more like watching grass grow. My development was gradual . . . a work in progress.

It's my theory that during this early period of uncertainty, almost all women come to hate themselves physically. I haven't met a woman yet who really likes her looks. That's because we don't identify with the finished product but with the anxious memory of waiting to see whether we'll win or lose. Not many draw a winning hand in the first round. But once the game begins, we can bluff our way through and play along the best we can. And that's the essence of the female persona, concentrating on our strong suit and shaping our hand into a winning streak.

How Do You Know If You're Pretty?

I didn't like my hair (very fine like my mother's), or my eyes (too deeply set and almond shaped, in standard-issue brown), or my nose (not cute enough), or my mouth (a bit too wide). Then there were my hips (not high or round enough) and my breasts (set too widely apart on my torso). But there were things I did like: my shoulders (square and broad), my back (shaped like an inverted triangle), and my waistline (super small). I also liked my skin (olive and fine-pored), my hands and feet (delicate and well-formed), and my teeth (super white, and I had my mother's smile). My cheekbones (prominent like Kate Hepburn's), my ears (small), and my proportions (svelte after years of ballet) were pretty damned good.

Looking around for confirmation, I wasn't able to spot anyone similar to my type whom I could gauge myself by. I judged myself "passable." Fortunately, any lack of confidence I had about my physical appeal wasn't shared by the opposite sex. They were not nearly as critical as I was. This became obvious from the way they stared at me when I got off the bus and walked down the street to my dance class. It was rather uncomfortable . . . but intoxicating.

Some guys would just gawk or drive around the block for a second look. But others would yell a lewd remark, make suggestive gestures and urge me to get in their car! It made me feel very exposed and vulnerable. "Go away!" was all I could think of to say; that, and zap them with an icy stare. After an awkward initiation period, I became accustomed and even immune to unwanted male attention. I was also flattered by the glances from other young girls who were sizing up the competition.

I didn't consider myself pretty, mainly because I didn't fit into the mold of the blonde, blue-eyed ideal. But who was I to argue? I rather liked being admired. At the same time, all the attention was distracting and interfered with the way I wanted to think of myself—as an intelligent girl with artistic leanings.

Windansea Beach

I enrolled in La Jolla High School, which was only three blocks away from the famous Windansea surfing beach! From the high school's second-story windows, my classmates could check out the coastline to see if the surf was up. Despite this siren call of the sea, once I enrolled as a freshman, I threw myself into my studies and managed to become an A student. Mr. Rosney, my all-time favorite teacher, taught American government, my best subject. I was keenly interested in Martin Luther King Jr. and his fight against racism and segregation. When it came to homework, I wasn't a fast reader, so I often had to work very late into the night to finish my assignments, sometimes until 3 AM. That didn't really bother me. I loved getting a handle on sociopolitical subjects. Whatever it took, I was ready to put forth the effort.

By now I had new idols. My parents didn't allow any movie fan magazines at our house. They were considered trash. But my best friend, Kitty Pemberton, had stacks of forbidden tabloids piled high all over her bedroom floor. We spent many an afternoon glued to the pages of those "rags." I pored over photos and stories about stars like Tony Curtis and Janet Leigh and couldn't get enough of James Dean, Natalie Wood, Jayne Mansfield, and Marilyn Monroe, as well as tons of starlets and teen idols.

Since the '90s, people have tended to refer to the '50s as an uptight period in our culture. I would argue with that perception. If that were true, how could this "squeaky clean" era have given rise to the world's most memorable sex symbols? Elvis Presley, Marilyn Monroe, James Dean, and Marlon Brando? They became my new idols. And they are still widely worshipped to this day.

Marilyn oozed "availability," which was how we young girls felt hormonally, though we had to put a lid on it. What troubled me back then was the fact that as hypnotic as Marilyn was to watch, she gave the impression of someone who could be easily taken advantage of and who couldn't fight back . . . like my mother. For that reason, I didn't want to be like her at all. She was an accident waiting to happen. Later, I saw that there were some men who could be protective. That was reassuring, but then they might end up taking ownership of you. Being a girl was like walking a tightrope. You just couldn't afford to walk with a wiggle.

And then came Elvis! It's amazing what his presence did to stimulate my teenage libido. Holy shit, he was something! I managed to get tickets to see him live at his first concert in the San Diego area. I sat eagerly waiting among thousands of screaming teenage girls when Elvis hit that stage. He was like a sexual hurricane, a force of nature. In reality, I didn't know the first thing about sex. But all of us sensed that Elvis had an irresistible grip on that subject. I can assure you that he had this fourteen-year-old girl "all shook up"!

Who could compete with Elvis? I had a record player stacked with 45s of "Heartbreak Hotel," "Jailhouse Rock," "Blue Suede Shoes," "Love Me Tender," and "Hound Dog." From that point on, something clicked in my head, and a new era was born. After that, I thought in terms of B.E. and A.E.: *Before Elvis* and *After Elvis*. He was a milestone. Until I met Jim Welch.

My First Love

James Wesley Welch was gorgeous. He had wavy black hair, green eyes, and a cool demeanor. I'll never forget the day I came running up the steps to my American government class and there he was. Whoa! Who's that? He looked at me and smiled his crooked grin. It was instant attraction. We were both fifteen. From the first minute I saw him, I secretly knew that I was destined to have his babies. In my emotionally charged, romantic young mind, I fixated on Jim as "my one and only."

He seemed to feel a magnetic pull toward me as well. Before long he asked if I wanted a ride to school, since he was one of the guys who had a car. He started picking me up in the morning and we'd drive to school together. I was in heaven. Jim would be my first true love, with all that it implies. He'd be the unforgettable, always present love, against whom all others would be judged. I couldn't even imagine that I would ever be in love with anyone else but him. That kind of *stinkin' thinkin'* would affect my personal life for years to come.

Love distracted me from my studies. I was always elated to see him and would chatter away nonsensically, out of sheer excitement. He, on the other hand, hardly said a thing! If he had, I might have discovered how little we had in common . . . but my schoolgirl crush on Jim lulled me into believing that he was the man of my dreams. And in some ways he was. And yet, I realized years later that I was needy and that it caused me to project certain qualities onto Jim that he didn't have.

Jim may not have talked very much, but he sure was a great dancer. We went to all the dances after the football games and jitter-bugged 'til we dropped! I had just become a cheerleader, and he was on the football team. Afterward, we'd pile into his car and head off to Oscar's Drive-in in Pacific Beach and have a burger and shake. It was the after-game hangout—very *American Graffiti*. Then we'd drive up to our favorite necking spot, Blueberry Hill (named after the Fats Domino song). It had a great view overlooking the village lights. It was just Jim and me and the radio.

Like most boys in my class, Jim drank beer; but I never touched the stuff. I just didn't like the taste. And it's a good thing, because during those sessions on "the Hill" when we were alone together, somebody had to draw the line. God knows, it was difficult. I just wanted to stay with him forever and never go home. Our song was "You Send Me," by Sam Cooke, one of my all-time favorites.

Jim represented the handsome young prince I had fantasized would rescue me. He was the antidote to my harsh father. Here was a young man who didn't ask anything much of me but showered me with the affection I was hungry for. But I couldn't cross the line and be intimate with him. I couldn't break the taboo.

I wasn't a Miss Goody Two-Shoes. None of the girls were "easy" back then. That's just the way it was among the girls in my school, who made up the class of 1958. Most of us were virgins, and I was no exception. Sex just wasn't discussed, and drugs were not in the picture. Porn was nowhere to be seen. *The Outlaw*, starring Jane Russell, was considered a very risqué movie, and no one under the age of twenty-one was allowed to see it. Eleven o'clock was the curfew. Daddy would be waiting up with the lights on when we pulled up. And Jim had better walk me to the door, or else!

Repressive? Maybe. But most girls respected the rules. The rules kept us in line, even though they would inevitably be broken. If you have no rules, you have no standards. Somehow, we all managed to get through high school without *acting out* the scenarios that were going on inside our heads. I feel that I was lucky that things were not more permissive. Looking back, I'm glad that I was reined in enough to take it slow in those formative years, if you call what happened in my life "slow." But it moved at a snail's pace by today's standards.

Although there was a lot of swooning and moaning, Jim and I weren't very sophisticated about sex. We were just all hot and bothered around each other. But during our third year of courtship, there were signs that we were also very different people. We kept breaking up and getting back together again. By our senior year, Jim, who never took much interest in his classes, dropped out of high school altogether. I was devastated! I had just become an honors student when he bailed and went off on a tuna clipper to Peru! I thought I'd never see him again. I knew that he'd been brooding about something, but it had never occurred to me that he would make such a drastic move. I didn't understand. Once he was gone, all I felt was hurt and confusion. I later realized that he needed to find himself and that academia was not his path. My father said, "Good riddance," and predicted that he'd never amount to anything. But I was brokenhearted and cried myself to sleep on many nights. Still, life went on.

High Heels and Bathing Suits

Only a year earlier, my life had taken an unexpected turn. It was one of those nonsensical things that happens and somehow changes everything. One day, out of the blue, I got talked into joining a beauty contest. My home economics teacher recruited all the girls in her class to participate as models at a photography convention. As part of this "field trip," we would also compete in a contest for the title "Miss Photogenic."

Huh? It had come out of left field, and I balked. We were being asked to wear one-piece bathing suits and high heels, of all things. I really didn't want to go. High heels and bathing suits sounded kind of cheesy to me, and I said so. But all the other girls thought I was trying to wriggle out of it and sort of shamed me into going along for the ride. So despite my grumbling, about a dozen of us ended up in Balboa Park one Sunday afternoon as models and rather unwilling contestants.

There were about 150 girls in the pageant from all over the city. What a big deal our glorified field trip had turned out to be. It was quite a scene backstage, with all of us primping and posing and stumbling about in heels. Before long I discovered that I actually liked to strut around in a pair of high heels and a bathing suit. It was fun! And because of the ballet, I was quite good at it. Those heels sure gave a girl tons of attitude. In the end, I walked off with the trophy.

Monday morning, the school campus was abuzz. My picture started appearing in the local papers, and complete strangers began to recognize me! It was my first taste of small-town fame, and it was exhilarating! But when the adrenaline stopped pumping, there was a bitter aftertaste. Even my friends treated me differently.

My win kicked off a series of events. Now the town council wanted me to enter the Miss La Jolla pageant. That was one I really wanted to win. After I became Miss La Jolla, I was automatically obligated to represent La Jolla in the countywide competition for Miss San Diego—the Fairest of the Fair. It was the beginning of a long line of beauty contests that eventually led to the state title of Maid of California. This was too much of a good thing. I was so done with all that . . . or so I thought.

That same year, I graduated with honors and received a scholarship to study theater arts at San Diego State College, where I also joined a sorority. But my heart wasn't in it. I couldn't stop thinking about Jim. I wondered when and if he would ever come home. He wrote to me from Peru, but his letters took forever to arrive. His mother, Tahnee Land, was always very sweet to me and kept me posted.

Months later, when Jim finally did come back home, I couldn't wait to see him. There I was, along with his mother and three sisters — Jan, Jerry, and Judy—waiting dockside to watch his ship come in. The Portuguese tuna clipper ambled sluggishly into sight looking like anything but a pleasure cruiser. But when I spotted Jim on deck, he was quite a sight for sore eyes. He was all tan and lean and muscled up from pulling those giant tuna nets aboard. He had also grown a rather dashing goatee and looked, for all the world, like John Derek in a pirate movie. Well, it was all over for me. I kept thinking what beautiful children we could make together. And I got my way. I dropped out of college, and we were married in Las Vegas. His mother, Tahnee, was there with us at the ceremony. We had her blessing. My mother was less than thrilled. My father was furious!

By marrying Jim, I was doing something for my own personal satisfaction and pretty much in defiance of my father's wishes. What I didn't anticipate was how a series of events would dovetail together and forever complicate my life. Jim and I were just settling into an apartment together and tackling the realities of married life: he was looking for a job, and I was calling my mother ten times a day for recipes and tips on cleaning products. However, my string of beauty titles was still generating enough heat and momentum to land me a regular stint on the local news channel, KFMB in San Diego, as the weather girl. It was a popular morning show called *Sun Up* and a great opportunity I didn't want to miss. So I didn't mind that I had to rise and shine each morning at 5 AM and leave early to tape the show.

Then, while I was still learning on the job how to report on the barometric pressure and describe cold fronts for the morning news, I started waking up to bouts of morning sickness! What a shock! That wasn't much fun. It was only a few months into the marriage and—bam!—I became pregnant, first with my son, Damon, and two years later with my daughter, Tahnee. Needless to say, Dad was even more pissed off than ever, and a period of estrangement between us kicked in.

I had dreams of using the recent exposure I'd gathered to start building an acting career, but now I could feel my resolve was crumbling. A girl can't live on professional ambitions alone. I hadn't counted on this unexpected turn. In fact, no one had anticipated where my strong emotional attachment to Jim would lead, and most of my inner circle was shocked to see my plans go so far off course. But at the heart of my feminine soul

I still felt that we were destined to be together. It would take more than a little nausea to shake my commitment. I had to see this thing through. And, happily, we had two adorable, healthy children. In fact, even my father's heart softened when he finally saw them. It was love at first sight.

Some might look at our union as a dreadful mistake. I used to think so myself at times, but in the final analysis it was truly a blessing. I knew that I had a decision to make. Was I to focus on my relationship with Jim and make a life with him, or was I to follow my ambitions for a career? The feminism of the '60s hadn't hit yet, but that didn't matter. I had never thought of asking for a consensus to follow my own mind, heart, and gut. Those were my willful days. The result was I had my first child at nineteen.

Even so, the birth of my two children had stopped me cold, and it took me a while to regain my equilibrium. I was forced to take a step back and reassess my whole life. Only it wasn't just mine anymore; it was ours. I still imagined that Jim and I could move forward together, with our children, but that was not to be.

Is Helen Gurley Brown's promise of "having it all" an idle one? Under the circumstances then, how could I hope for that? How could I be true to my biological destiny and my loving feminine nature and also not defect from my personal calling? As things evolved, opportunities did come a-knocking from Hollywood, but I wanted to go to New York and do theater. However, Jim had his own ideas, and unfortunately they didn't include either option for me. The breach that grew between us over the next few years gave me the license to gather up my two kids and leave my hometown and my marriage behind. But I didn't make it to New York. Moving to the Big Apple was an expensive proposition and with two children would prove too difficult. I had started to save money from modeling jobs for the airfare, but my locker at work was broken into and my money stolen. This setback was too much for me. I took it as an omen and changed my destination to Los Angeles, where at least I wouldn't have to acquire an entirely new wardrobe for four different seasons and worry about where my kids would play. As a Southern California girl, I didn't even own a winter coat.

My breakup with Jim remains the most painful decision of my entire life. For our children's sake, I should have stayed. Kudos to my mother on that score. C. S. Lewis wrote that you "stand taller when you bow." But I wasn't in the bowing mood. People talk about "falling in love," but there is also a *will* to love, which is what it all boils down to after the honeymoon is over. At our painfully young age, we didn't have the serious relationship tools to manage that kind of love. Those qualities come with a maturity that I couldn't even dream of possessing at the time. We were both just too damn young.

That doesn't, however, excuse me. The damage I did to my children and Jim by taking off as I did is immeasurable. It would take a whole book to get into it. I have no defense for my foolishness, except to say that I was young and pigheaded. My children are the best thing in my life . . . that I *haven't* done. Their good character, resourcefulness, and talents are all to their own credit. More on that subject later, when I can delve a bit further into motherhood.

Mommy Takes Hollywood

Flash forward only three short years, on the heels of my breakup with Jim and the beginning of my struggles in Hollywood. When I got there, with no car, two hundred bucks in my pocket, two kids, and no connections, it was pretty rough going. I ran into all kinds of weirdness. For one thing, children were considered personae non gratae back then. It was difficult to even rent an apartment. In early 1963, 90 percent of the vacancy signs specified "No Children." A couple of toddlers were not the kind of baggage a young actress starting out could advertise around town. It was wise to keep a low profile.

All of it was hateful and demoralizing. But I knew I was just passing through, and I didn't need the acceptance of those who disapproved. I just held my nose and gave myself a make-or-break, three-year deadline. Sometimes even today I drive by the first apartment we stayed in, just as a reminder of what a miracle it is that we survived that wicked period. What doesn't kill you makes you stronger. My early experience in H'wood vaccinated me against sleaze and phonies.

When I hit town, it was all about Bond, *James Bond*, and I almost became a Bond girl! I was tested for *Thunderball*. Producer Cubby Broccoli had seen my photo in a *Life* magazine layout called "The End of the Great Girl Drought!" He called Jack Gilardi, my agent at GAC, and the subsequent buzz around town created so much excitement that it enabled me to bag a long-term contract at 20th Century Fox. But because of a technicality involving start dates and contract options, Fox put me in the sci-fi classic *Fantastic Voyage*. I was disappointed. Here I was ready to snuggle up to Sean Connery but was assigned to eight months floating through the human bloodstream in a wet suit instead.

Since the '60s, sexy girls always seem to end up in sci-fi features; and they're still doing it. Look at Jessica Alba and Megan Fox. Since I was still unproven at the time, I was hoping that Fox would groom me for more challenging roles. But as fate would have it, the studio had a completely different plan for me. My first starring role was to be in a dinosaur epic called *One Million Years B.C.* Fox's studio head, Dick Zanuck, called to tell me that I would be playing the part of Loana in this remake of the 1940 caveman classic. Although I thanked him for my "big break," all I could think was, *A dinosaur movie? You've got to be kidding me!* I figured my performance would disappear without a trace.

Four brief months later came the release of the poster for *One Million Years B.C.* Several million copies of that image were circulated throughout the planet to herald the launch of the movie. And now we've come full circle to the moment you probably first became aware of me.

There I was, staring out at the world as though from the beginning of time. The cultural critic Camille Paglia later described it as "the indelible image of a woman as queen of nature. She was a lioness: fierce, passionate and dangerously physical." Anyway, the doeskin bikini struck a chord. I became every male's fantasy.

In the photograph, I look so convincing, so formidable standing there astride the rocky landscape in that partially shredded animal skin. I seem alert and slightly defiant, as though ready to defend myself against anyone who might attempt to tear the mini-toga off me. Or like a mama bear, ready to protect her cubs.

In one way the image was very apt, because I knew I was going to have to fight to stay afloat in the most treacherous of identities: the role of sex symbol. There I was, stranded and easy prey in that desolate realm of overnight success. But I was nobody's pushover. Would I be just a flash in the pan, as some predicted? It was me against the world. Or should I say *us*, if you count my two children. When that famous photo was snapped on location, my little ones were miles away, playing by the hotel pool with their nanny at the bottom of a mountain, while Mom was atop a smoking volcano . . . and it was snowing!

In fact, it was *soooo* cold that the entire crew was bundled up in nice cozy parkas. Even the cameras froze. So they hung pots of hot coals underneath the camera boxes, to keep the motors warm. But nobody seemed to care about *my* motor. Why didn't I have a parka? "Cave girls don't have parkas," I was told. Not surprisingly, I came down with a severe case of tonsillitis.

It was *so* not how I had pictured it. On the first day of shooting, I went straight up to the director, Don Chaffey, and said quite seriously, "Listen Don, I've been studying the script, and I was thinking . . ." He turned to me in amazement and said, "*You* were thinking? Don't." Then he said, "You see that rock over there?" I was all ears. "That's Rock A. When I call action, you start running all the way over to Rock B, which is over there. When you get about midway between the two, pretend you see a giant turtle coming over that hill. You scream . . . and we break for lunch. Got it?"

I got it all right. He was just the first in a long line of producers and directors who didn't give a rat's ass what I thought. For years I felt like the Rodney Dangerfield of sex symbols. I got no respect.

I'm glad those days are over. But I was wrong about the dinosaur movie; it wasn't a leap into obscurity. By the time we wrapped and I boarded a flight for London, unbeknownst to me, my life was already changing. When I stepped off the plane in Heathrow Airport, I was greeted by a swarm of press and paparazzi. What was the deal? No one could be more surprised by this than I was! Suddenly, I had become famous! I had to pinch myself. Was it really happening? It was a once-in-a-lifetime break for me and my kids.

So Mommy became the reigning sex symbol of the swingin' '60s and '70s, at the height of the sexual revolution—with one hitch. A sex symbol in the Age of Flower Children didn't sit very well with the hard-line feminists of the time. They dismissed me as nothing more than a sex object. They didn't look beyond the poster image to see what I was made of. It felt like a slap, until I realized that official feminism had a political agenda that is not inclusive of all women. It's only for those who fit a criterion, which does not include a bikini. So be it.

I don't want to fall into the cliché of the protesting sex symbol, but I have to supply a context so you know who it is that's talking to you here. Although this book is not intended to be an autobiography, I feel the need to let you in on who is lurking behind the loincloth. It's me, Raquel: a woman not unlike you in many ways and singular in others. Like we all are. Hello there! Nice to meet you.

In the movie *The Shawshank Redemption*, my poster from *One Million Years B.C.* was one of a series of posters used to cover the escape tunnel Tim Robbins was digging. I was flattered when the director, Frank Darabont, asked permission to use my image to represent the passage of time from Rita Hayworth in the '40s to Marilyn Monroe in the '50s to Raquel Welch in the '60s.

In the film, it takes Robbins twenty-odd years to dig himself out of captivity and into freedom. There were times when I wondered if I, too, would ever dig myself out from behind that image and into the liberating light of day. But I've grown fond of my former alter ego—cave girl Loana. She and I get along just fine now. After all, we're basically different sides of the same personality. And if I ask her nicely, she steps aside and gets out of my way. Nevertheless, the loincloth is in mothballs now. When I look back at that poster today, I have to smile and say, "Who is she?"

After our marriage crashed and burned, Jim got drafted and joined the Green Berets. Once separated, we ended up in two different worlds and we lived continents apart. For a number of reasons, including the distance, our work demands and bruised feelings, Jim and I didn't confer directly for an extended period of time. My mother or sister would pass messages between us. As a result, the children only visited with their father intermittently for a while. It was far from ideal, and I blame myself for allowing that.

I carried on with my career and remarried three more times. I made more than forty-five feature films, tackled Broadway musicals, and had my successes. Jim became a multimillionaire real estate developer. He's married, and he and his wife Jean have a son, Jonas. Damon and Tahnee now enjoy a close relationship with their father, and he and I have been on very friendly terms for decades.

Fortunately, my children and I have a good relationship, and they're still my great joy. My son, Damon, became a computer consultant engineer, and my daughter, Tahnee, a talented actress known for her role in *Cocoon*. They are a source of pride and hope to me because of the kind of people they've turned out to be. They have always grounded me and given me purpose, as well as the moral courage to follow my better convictions. Now if they'll just give me grandchildren, I'll be complete. That's an ambition of mine only they can fulfill.

I should add that, at my present age, with the luxury of hindsight, I've noticed a tendency in my gender to underestimate the value of being a member of the female sex. I've fought that tendency in myself, and have come to adopt a more positive and empowering attitude toward *the art of being a woman.*

And as for you, dear reader, I hope that some of my backstory has brought us closer together. Now that you know a little more about me and how I evolved as a woman, let's move ahead.

TWO

The Art of Being a Woman ... at Any Age

"I'M A WOMAN ... W-O-M-A-N!" TO QUOTE
the words of that sassy Peggy Lee song. And I decided long ago that
it's far better to master what I call the art of being feminine, feline, and
female and everything that goes with girlishness, rather than to resent
and ultimately resist my biological destiny. I have banished any regrets
related to being a member of "the weaker sex."

Every woman has a choice to make. We either embrace the special power and, yes, the magic of being a woman, or forever live a life
of discontent. The irony is that 90 percent of the so-called "stronger sex"
spends the better part of their lives in the act of pursuing us, winning
our favor and trying their best — if you'll excuse the expression — to get
laid. Women are what makes the world go 'round, and that's not a job
for sissies.

Out of deference to all the "libbers" out there — I'm a lapsed lib-
ber myself — I have to cop to wrestling with my own frustration over the
inequities of being born female. As you already know, I, too, had to
overcome some pretty big anger issues with my father and learn to forgive and forget. It wasn't easy.

I do believe that, in a sense, facing up to my challenging relationship with my father in my teens gave me a more accepting attitude. It

helped me find a place in my heart to be more forgiving of men and to understand the perennial battle between the sexes. It seems to me that, if you see men as the enemy, you merely want to annihilate them for their cocky sense of entitlement. But if you see men as your true partners in life—though necessarily different from you—you've got a shot at putting up with some of the maddening foolishness and meanness that characterizes some of their less-than-ideal behavior. Though we have to admit, it's really a pretty even trade-off, considering some of our female antics, which are downright spiteful . . . PMS hysterics, anyone?

The machismo of the classic man—a dying breed—and his street-smart swagger may annoy us at times. But it's often merely a front to protect the fragile male ego. A man needs to present himself as invulnerable and able to "handle" the competition in *any* situation. Bring it on! Men face some formidable challenges and frankly don't have the wiggle room or options many women do. They usually aren't given the choice between having a vocation and being "a house husband." Supporting a family and earning a substantial living is still considered the measure of a man.

As a matter of fact, little has changed for men through the ages. It's *man*datory that he succeed as a provider and compete in the workplace. In addition, his physical stature and toughness are constantly under scrutiny, and not just in sports. His social skills and intellectual capacity are tested and crucial to attracting a woman. We complain a lot about typical male behavior, yet don't take into account that a man needs to uphold his reputation on all fronts, inspiring respect and confidence wherever he goes, especially among "the ladies."

John Wayne was the perfect example of the "manly man." He was willing and able to take on anything and anybody . . . including the fiery Maureen O'Hara. But in today's world, pleasing a woman isn't exactly a slam dunk. Male anxiety in the boudoir is epidemic, owing to the demands of legions of lovelies whose performance standards are higher than ever. They don't expect to be disappointed sexually . . . nor is once enough! It's almost as if there's an applause meter hanging over her bed. No wonder Viagra sales are booming! I pity those men who don't fit comfortably into their role and aren't the ideal Gladiator, Cowboy, Astronaut, Godfather, James Bond or Master of the Universe.

I feel for them, but here's the rub: every morning a guy wakes up and zooms through the three S's—sh*t, shower, and shave—and afterward he's ready to roll. A woman, on the other hand, has to face a laundry list of daily, some might say superficial, demands, including but not limited to doing her hair (complete with curling iron, flat iron and blow dryer all crowded into one beleaguered wall socket). I don't know how any couple manages to "share" a bathroom!

Then there's the task of putting on makeup, coordinating an outfit (shoes, handbag, jewelry, a wrap), and making sure you change what you're wearing every day—and don't repeat an outfit too often. And all this on a budget, in most cases! Finally, we have to emerge from this exacting ritual in good humor, with a smiling face and a lilt to our voice, regardless of whether or not we're having a bad hair day.

Now add to that menstrual cramps, bloating, and emotional swings wide enough to rival an acrobat from Cirque du Soleil; plus the grind of staying in shape to fulfill all those male fantasies; while also pursuing a career or a given talent. Then there's the agony of falling in love; being a lover, wife, daughter, sister, and friend; creating a warm and loving home; giving birth (no need to get too graphic here); and, of course, the awesome responsibility of motherhood.

Peggy Lee got it right when she reeled off the list:

> *I can wash out forty-four pair of socks*
> *And have 'em hangin' out on the line*
> *Feed the baby, grease the car, and powder my nose*
> *All at the same time*

Let's face it, there ain't *nothin'* a sister can't do! But is it righteously fair? Don't look for fair.

Ah . . . to be born a woman and to try to live up to the expectations! The worst part is simply coming to grips with what womanhood demands without getting discouraged. It's a spectacular part—I mean, you wouldn't want anything less, would you? You didn't want to get stuck in a minor role, did you? This gives you a chance to flaunt *all* your talents. It's an opportunity to shine! Who else could enable, nurture, appease, inspire, and spread the feeling to others that life is worth living. That's why God created woman!

One thing for sure, it's all part of the divine scheme of things, verified since the beginning of time by the ancient use of symbolism. Man and woman are complementary sides of the same coin *and*, accordingly, related to all the essential elements in the world. The sun is masculine and the moon feminine. The sea of life is a woman (*la mer* in French), while the captain of the ship is masculine. A man sails his vessel through the waves, carving out a course for himself in the vast ocean. The Latin word for man is *vir*, associated with *virtus*, which means "virtue" and is associated with manly courage and virility. I love to think of it this way . . . we are the sea, girls. We can rock his world!

Fortunately, there's never a dull moment. Yes, we're entitled to grumble and moan under our breath. But when the time comes, I favor trying my best to be a good sport and refraining from whining. I enjoy playing my hand and having a blast.

How to make a man happy and have him return the favor? Well, to borrow a phrase from one of my favorite actresses, and a feisty one at that: "Fasten your seat belts, it's going to be a bumpy night." Let's not forget, the poor guys are jumping through hoops for our benefit. If they're not, your standards aren't high enough.

Some Things Are Better Left Unsaid!

Before I get too carried away here, I should qualify my fervor and make clear that I do *not* define myself *solely* by my relationship with the opposite sex. At the same time, I refuse to deny my feminine nature and acknowledge that the way I move through life and my methods of making a contribution rest on my femininity. I rely on my feminine strength and resilience, which is, I've discovered, quite different from masculine strength, both mentally and physically. We are not wired the same.

There are women out there who are less tied to their feminine side than I am, and I have no problem with them. But sometimes I feel they disapprove of women who are ultra feminine. I try to be more inclusive. I think we all have something different to bring to the table. We don't have to fit into the same mold, with one exception.

For professional women, like myself, there's a danger of confusing equality of the sexes with sameness. Trying to "act like" a man only undermines your strengths as a woman and plays into the "bitch" syndrome. Yes, I've been there, done that, too. Not anymore. Which doesn't mean you shouldn't stand up for yourself when the occasion arises. But watch your mouth. Men, especially, don't listen to a word you say, but they pay rapt attention to the tone in which you say it. Talking tough doesn't help; that's their territory.

Finding the balance between being a strong, capable woman and a ballbreaker is the dilemma facing most of us on a daily basis—both in business and at home. Female pride is a good thing, but real girl power is making others—including men—feel important and good about themselves. You don't have to *fake it*, you just need to see things from their perspective in order to really understand them. And if *that* doesn't work . . . go ahead and fake it.

It has been said, "By your words you will be known." So choose your words carefully, remembering that when you lose your poise, you lose your power. And that, by the way, goes for discussing sexually related subjects as well.

One has to wonder about the legacy of the '60s wave of sexual freedom, which I experienced first hand. Once women started applauding themselves for "talking openly about sex" and the reproductive process, there was no end to it. They couldn't shut up. The floodgates were thrown open, and so were women's legs. There's something about the spoken word that is as potent as a bullet. It can be lethal. Saying the wrong thing can cause a lot of permanent damage to yourself and others. And women usually diffuse their purpose by talking *too much*. Girlfriend, there's a time when certain things are better left unsaid.

Our entire culture is so preoccupied with sex, you can't avoid the trash talk, but you don't have to contribute to it. Oh, I know you'll gossip with friends and can cuss like a sailor on occasion, but there's still something to be said about *sounding* like a lady in public. Yet, it never ceases to amaze me when the more intellectual, cultured and accomplished women of our time find it necessary to contribute to a post-feminist obsession with politicizing sex. Some feel compelled to participate in performance events and public readings that I refer to as *labia chic*.

Case in point: My phone rang one afternoon back in the early '90s with an offer to appear in *The Vagina Monologues*. As I read this critically acclaimed work with A-list endorsements, I was confronted with page after page of graphic gynecological jargon, which should be confined to the realm of pelvic exams with both feet in the stirrups! Yikes! Is this supposed to be relevant feminism? I wondered. It was definitely not my cup of tea. We've come a very long way, baby . . . but in which direction? Has the culmination of feminist progress led to this moment? I fail to see how talking to your vagina can elevate a woman's self-esteem. I'd sooner mail a letter through that slot. Don't misunderstand me, I recognize that this play was written to deliver a political message and to address painful issues of shame afflicting some women, but it's the choice of method I take exception to. There's a reason why God put the female apparatus *inside* the body.

Sure, guys obsess aloud about the size of their organs and their sexual prowess and boast about the notches on their guns. I say let them, if they must. Men remain little boys their entire lives, with their hands on their crotches. Women need not become vulgar in an effort to imitate men. A real sister remains above all that. Cross your legs, girls! Guard that womb. What ever happened to mystery?

And now for the obligatory disclaimer: No, I'm not frigid, sexually frustrated, prudish, or unfulfilled. But if this is the new hip, I wanna be square.

The problem for today's younger women is that most have lowered their standards so drastically that societal expectations have also sunk along with them. Among the decent, admirable, honest, hardworking mothers and young professional women of the YouTube generation, the public spotlight has been captured by a new breed of *sexhibitionists*, who have become role models for a distressing number of prepubescent girls. When did a mug shot become a prerequisite for fame? *Girls Gone Wild* has unfortunately become the prototype for recreational sex. And while cheers of "you go, girl" echo from the sidelines, young women are being reduced to disposable sex toys.

Looking back over my own early years, I now realize that I was fortunate to spend my youth being protected. Whether at home or at school, I was closely supervised by authority figures: parents, teachers, the codes of behavior that extended to school corridors, and even by public airwaves and the popular media, which used to steer clear of smut. I grew up in a time when the national media was not rife with sexual images and four-letter words were not signaled with a bleep. They simply weren't allowed. I'm not suggesting that we revert to those times. But if things *had been different* and sexed-up when I was a kid, it might have persuaded me away from the limits my parents had laid down for me. Back then, no one was conversing with their sexual organs . . . at least not in public. I was *protected by my environment*. The whole of society was youth friendly, *not by overindulgence, but by discipline and, most importantly, by setting an example*. Now we are more concerned about polluting the environment than we are about the pollution of young minds.

Not far from the turn of the new millennium, it has become painfully clear to me exactly where a certain stripe of feminism has taken us. I hate to say it, but the main thing that resonates today out of Hippie Feminism is the sexual revolution and its promise of better orgasms. By then, fortunately, I was already past puberty and the movement toward sexual freedom wasn't pivotal to my early development. I already had my moral foundations in place and knew enough to quietly fend for myself against social pressure. How does today's kind of public endorsement of premarital sex and ridicule of virgins affect the behavior and identity of very young girls and women? In a later chapter I'd like to delve more deeply into this question and the role feminism played in sexuality for women of all ages. It's a complicated subject, but pivotal to our daughters and their future.

In recent years, after speaking engagements for AARP and various women's groups of the boomer-plus generation, I've come away with a warm, familial sense that we have all been in the trenches together. We share a common history, and though your experiences may have been different from mine, it still follows that we have in our separate ways crossed similar bridges and faced — perhaps not the same — but parallel fears and challenges.

It must have been a woman who coined the phrase, "diamond in the rough." It reminds me of the way I view myself when I look in the mirror. On first glance I don't see beauty . . . I only see possibilities. It's a good metaphor for the art of being a woman; we are like unrefined raw material that on the surface doesn't reveal its true value until it's mined, cut, and polished to perfection. The catch is that just when you have mastered this bit of feminine alchemy and finally gotten your act together . . . you're facing forty!

THREE

Forty and Beyond

AGE FORTY DOES *NOT* PACK THE SAME WALLOP
it once did. Not all of us today look upon our fortieth year with the same
trepidations our mothers did. And judging by the Facebook generation
(1995 through 2010), hitting forty is destined to become even less significant. Unfortunately, however, the negative undertones regarding aging still remain, threatening to cut short our opportunities prematurely.

When I hit forty, I'd long been part of the fitness revolution.
Women had begun to share athleticism freely with men. As a result, a
large percentage of us had not aged at the same rate as the previous generation of women had. Physically at least, forty had almost lost its bite!
I viewed my fortieth birthday as cause for celebration, and I began making plans to announce it publicly to the media. It seemed like a good idea
at the time. *Not!* In Hollywood, such a confession is more like career sui-
cide! I was about to come nose to nose with a nasty little reality called
ageism. And it wasn't pretty. In the dog-eat-dog entertainment industry, with its attendant media scrutiny, forty still marks a point when the
first barbed references to age start to pollute the atmosphere, accompanied by whispered insinuations that the axe is about to fall. Maybe
you know the feeling? Even those of us who are not in the public eye

have experienced the dread of being rejected or diminished by an arbitrary number.

Is forty too old? Definitely *not*, and I stand by that. It seems to me that forty is the age when a woman reaches her physical and mental peak. When I entered that fateful year, an entire generation of women, who like me were born on the eve of a World War II victory, were also experiencing the same sense of coming into their own. We were bred on Elvis Presley and the intoxicating birth of rock 'n' roll. We were architects of an irreverent generation that changed the world in the '60s! We burned our bras and started the celebrated counterculture and sexual revolution. We were the men and women who invented the Generation Gap. The only problem is . . . now we're in it! The youth culture is unquestionably our legacy, but in our attempt to break with the restrictions and traditions of the past, have we thrown the baby out with the bathwater?

Today the O-word is the new profanity, and no one is immune. It's the only dirty word left in the English language. Nowadays you can call a woman a ho, a porno slut, a ball-breaker, a dyke, an endless array of four-letter words, but don't risk calling her the O-word! Even men are running scared. Everyone over forty is terrified of being called "old," and that's just the tip of the iceberg. Respect for our elders and people of experience was completely trashed during the '60s. Now it's gone.

Why do Americans feel it necessary to expel or *segregate* such a huge segment of the population from the mainstream? Except as pharmaceutical consumers, boomers don't seem to exist . . . all 75 million of us! What are they smoking? We, who show such compassion for animals and the environment, seem barely fazed by the isolation of a vast portion of the population over the age of fifty. What a waste! If, like me, you're over sixty, that isolation becomes even more intense. Plus, it sets in motion a boomerang effect that will return to afflict future generations, who in turn will have to suffer the consequences of the very same cold shoulder as they age.

Here's the bottom line: when we get past forty, it's a minefield out there. We have no choice but to wage psychological warfare with a media that conspires to discount and ignore us, because we are not as easy to manipulate as a younger and more gullible demographic. This focus on the youth market makes experienced and discerning adults obsolete in their, or should I say our, prime.

In my opinion, forty should be a time of celebration. I think it's precisely the moment when a woman finally feels comfortable in her own skin. And yet, terms like "preferred demographics," invented by the advertising world, seek to define which consumers manufacturers should direct their marketing toward. They cater almost exclusively to a certain age group, discarding the boomer-plus generation as undesirable. Talk about profiling!

Confronting Ageism

I stopped lying about my age when I turned forty. I was emboldened by the notion that, by 1980, forty was no longer the critical turning point in a woman's life it was once advertised to be. I could have easily lied about my age and gotten away with it, but that would have meant surrendering to my most fearful impulses. After wrestling with this decision, I came to the conclusion that my dread of what the truth might cost me far surpassed the reality of the situation. So, like David facing Goliath with his slingshot, I opted to launch my fortieth year with a splash. Despite the repercussions that might result, I hoped to slay the threat of this milestone and transform it into a joyful rite of passage.

The timing couldn't have been better. World-famous fashion photographer Victor Skrebneski was planning to shoot me as the subject of an elaborate black-and-white photo exhibit at the prestigious Richard Gray Gallery, in my birthplace of Chicago, thus providing the perfect occasion to celebrate my fortieth birthday! I realize in retrospect that it was a nervy thing to do. Hollywood sex symbols *do not* celebrate turning forty! It's a big no-no.

Was I wrong to come out of the closet about my age? Let's examine this for a moment. If people thought I was younger, why tell them otherwise? I'd been exposed to the theory that "perception *is* reality." This is a conceit that has nothing to do with the truth. But much of the media operates on the premise that if something is repeated often enough, it *becomes* true, because *most people don't form their own opinions.* They tend to adopt whatever mind-set is out there as their own and go along for the ride. Like it or not, the public is often led around by the nose. I call it brainwashing by consent! So for me, backing away from my fortieth year seemed like selling out.

The spectacular photo exhibit in Chicago, in combination with my fortieth-birthday announcement, was a big success! I felt vindicated!

The Turning Point

Unfortunately, that very year, 1980, my age was the reason cited for my dismissal from the cast of the MGM movie *Cannery Row*, in which I was set to star opposite Nick Nolte. The movie was based on two John Steinbeck novels, *Cannery Row* and *Sweet Thursday.* I sued MGM for wrongful termination, and when the case was tried in court, I found myself characterized as an over-the-hill actress playing a part I was too old for. I had been cast in the role of Suzy, who has come to Cannery Row to get a job in Monterey during the Depression. When that fails, she ends up working at a cathouse as one of "the girls," out of desperation. One would have thought I was age appropriate to play opposite Nick Nolte, who falls for my character, Suzy. And I was part of a pool of actresses being considered that included Julie Christie, Jessica Lange, and Jane Fonda, most of whom were my age or close to it. Nick was playing the part of a marine biologist, Doc (an alter ego of Steinbeck himself), who frequented this same house of ill repute. The idea was that opposites attract . . . the scientist and the hooker.

In the end I was replaced by the much younger actress, Debra Winger. I don't feel any of this was at all her fault, but was the work of MGM studio head David Begelman, who had been indicted a few years earlier in an embezzlement scandal at Columbia Studios. (Academy Award–winning actor Cliff Robertson was responsible for bringing that case to light and was blacklisted as a result.) Although Begelman had approved my casting, he didn't flinch from using my age as an excuse for removing me from the movie and ignoring my pay-or-play contract. The fallout from his actions in my case caused the virtual end of my film career.

Artistically speaking, I felt that because of my maturity I was on the threshold of doing my best work as an actress, and was anticipating this chance to sink my teeth into a meaty role. So when this devastating turn of events took place, it hit me hard.

On the advice of my attorneys, I attempted to reach a settlement with the studio, hopeful that they would reassign me to another movie and thereby undo the damage done by "yanking" me out of *Cannery Row*. Begelman and MGM refused, leaving me no alternative but to sue them for nonpayment and damaging my professional reputation. This was a very dangerous move on my part. I would be bucking the male-dominated system. In the end, I felt I had to stand up for myself and clear my name.

During the course of the trial, my lawyers subpoenaed all the footage that had been shot of me in the role of Suzy. When the judge and jury finally viewed those scenes, the consensus was that not one of the claims against me, including the concern over my age suitability, could be justified. It also raised the question of whether my dismissal had been premeditated.

As the court looked deeper into this issue, a conflict of interest came to light. Unbeknownst to me, my agent was *also* representing Debra Winger! I sat stunned as the evidence revealed a series of conspiratorial exchanges between the studio and my agent regarding Winger's availability. Apparently, a plan was afoot for Winger to step into my role once the picture was green lit and principal photography had begun. So that's how and why they "unloaded" me.

The upshot was that my phone did not ring for a full year after my dismissal. I had fallen off the planet of working actresses, and now I was on the outside looking in. So I went away with my husband at the time—French screenwriter André Weinfeld—to my favorite island of Mustique, to lick my wounds. On the way back we stopped in New York to see a friend, and it was there, just when prospects couldn't have looked bleaker, that I received an offer to appear on Broadway in the musical *Woman of the Year.* I took it gladly . . . throwing myself into rehearsals with full-bodied enthusiasm. It was my first time on the boards in the Big Apple, and I loved every minute of it! Luckily, my success in that role, which required me to sing, dance, and do smart comedy dialogue, jump-started interest in me—this time in a more legitimate way—and revitalized my career.

The impact of my debut on the Great White Way landed me on the covers of *Life* magazine and *Vanity Fair.* A television movie that I had produced for NBC before being cast in *Cannery Row* was broadcast and got a whopping 36 share, which represented huge ratings! Grant Tinker, head of the network, was over-the-moon happy. I was on a roll again. And yet, I could not get a motion picture agent and was not invited back into the good favor of the Hollywood community for several years to come. But everything happens for a reason . . . God does move in mysterious ways.

It took six long years for the case to get to court, during which I was extremely grateful for the friendship of Swifty and Mary Lazar and Cary Grant, as well as for letters of encouragement from Burt Reynolds and Burt Lancaster, who lent their moral support. Eventually, I won the case and was awarded $25,000,000—later reduced to $11,000,000 on appeal—for wrongful termination and for damage done to my film career. Though delighted to have won the lawsuit, I would have preferred to continue with my movie career, minus the bias that resulted from taking on the Hollywood system.

Even today, turning forty in Hollywood is no picnic, and it certainly made me vulnerable in a very cutthroat business. My only consolation is that when *Cannery Row* was released—without my forty-year-old presence—it opened and closed in three days! As the famed syndicated columnist and New York icon Liz Smith commented,

"Raquel Welch should send flowers to whoever was responsible for getting her out of this turkey!"

The Big Five-O

By some miracle, I managed to survive—even thrive—through my forties and was able to climb back on top again. But hot on its heels came my fifties! . . . and that's a horse of a different color. Even though we boomers are enjoying the luxury of a longer life and a more attractive and vital older age, the odds are no longer in our favor. Why? The "new age" executives have deemed us inadequate by an outdated measuring stick. And we feel the snub! We run the risk of being benched—pulled from the field of action and left to sit and watch from the sidelines. It affects our sense of self-worth and, even worse, stunts our meaningful contribution to a troubled culture that is sorely in need of our experience and input.

Granted, there are different stages in life, and I'm the first to admit that each has a different scenario, but this generation of fifty-plus boomers is breaking new ground. We have an obligation to show the younger generation by example—if by nothing else—how to navigate through an *extra twenty to thirty bonus years* of life! This extended longevity can prove to be a very fruitful and enjoyable period. But, led by Hollywood, advertisers and retailers seem convinced that Americans over fifty are too set in their buying habits and incapable of adapting to an ever-changing pop culture. *Au contraire*! Did they forget that boomers were the architects of the '60s? *Our religion is change.*

I don't know about you, but I hate to walk into a department store ready to spend and not be able to find anything that fits! They don't carry any sizes for real women, just for girls. Are you familiar with this predicament? I mean, I'm not a size 4 anymore, and by the way . . . is that a bra cup or an eggcup? Not only do retailers seem blind to our existence, they don't even seem interested in our money. Big mistake! Recently the Dove ad campaign and the buyers for department stores have shown signs of an awakening, but the culture has a long way to go. As for me, I'm not remotely ready to roll over and play dead yet. Are you?

We can all agree that aging is challenging, but believe me, it can be even more so for a fading sex symbol.

Everywhere I go, women in particular stop me to ask a slew of questions, assuming that I'm an expert on the subject of aging and I know *all* the answers. Ha! If only! What I do know, however, is that as a woman of a "certain age" I've had to adopt a new approach and a completely different attitude. Call it a newfound humility. As we grow older we have to accept that we are no longer in control. Actually, we never were . . . but we didn't realize it then. If you want to tackle the ravages of time and not look like a plastic surgery junkie or become a slave to denial, there's a lot to consider, vital choices to make and countless decisions to be put into play for your own preservation and sanity. No joke, getting older can be an absolute "beyotch"! But it doesn't *have* to be, if you play your cards right.

Part II

THE
HEALTHY
WOMAN

FOUR

Healthy Menopause

THERE'S NO QUESTION THAT THE BATTLE against aging truly begins in earnest at the crucial point of menopause. Up until then, all the fussing and obsessing about little flaws may loom large in the female consciousness, but once you start to enter the pre-menopausal or perimenopausal phase, you realize that your life will be irreversibly changed. In retrospect, everything leading up to that moment seems like a cakewalk to me.

The expression "change of life" is an understatement. Until I hit fifty, I was feeling pretty cocky. Then I hit a brick wall. The experience is different for every woman, but for me, fifty was the acid test. We're talkin' a serious breakdown in the hormonal system. I could almost feel the fountain of youth draining away . . . drip, by drip, by drip. It was a strange sensation that I know at least some of you have shared. It left such a vivid impression on me that if I close my eyes, I can almost recapture the precise moment when I felt myself fading into a mere shadow of my former self. Try it sometime. Go ahead, close your eyes. Can you feel it? Personally, I always imagine that when I open my eyes I'll be standing in a little pool of estrogen!

I'm well aware that there are some women who sail right through menopause, unfazed. I was not so lucky. The hot flashes were just the tip of the iceberg. My energy level took a major nosedive, and I was re-duced to tears every time I misplaced my keys. There were moments when I began to wonder if these nightmarish symptoms were some kind of sadistic payback for all those years I spent strutting around in a bikini.

I'd been doing so well up until then, but "the change" caught me off guard, like an ambush. No question about it. Fifty knocked me sideways!

I was an emotional wreck. Forget PMS . . . this was serious. Every little thing—like waking up in the morning—made me cry. I was aboard a wacky roller-coaster ride without a clue about how to make it stop.

Leading up to my first major episode, I had been in intensive train-ing for a television commercial for Crystal Light. The script called for me to wear a skintight bodysuit while performing a musical number. I'd be singing away and dancing along a narrow, elevated catwalk, and then exiting offstage to drink a refreshing glass of Crystal Light, a low-cal beverage for figure-conscious women. Normally, this would have been a snap for me. I didn't yet realize that I had entered a time in my life when my supply of hormones was diminishing. Before long, I noticed that when I worked out strenuously, which I'd been doing for most of my adult life, the loss of estrogen from the exertion now caused me to bleed a bit ("spotting"), much like the light days most women experi-ence at the beginning and end of their menstrual cycle. So I backed off on my workouts, because I was also feeling weak and tired. The spot-ting persisted. Every time I overextended myself to the slightest degree, it started up again. Somehow I got through the shoot, and nobody was the wiser. But I was worried.

I consulted my gynecologist, who told me after some blood tests that I was perimenopausal, which meant entering the menopause phase, and that I should keep him posted. He confirmed that every woman is different, and my symptoms were specific to me.

My next professional commitment was another body-conscious

gig. This time, it was an exercise video for HBO, with whom I had a contract to produce a library of four Raquel Welch fitness videos. I had already done three videos after my Broadway debut in *Woman of the Year*, and this was to be my fourth. Once again, a week or two into training, I found myself losing stamina, and sure enough, I started "spotting" again, but this time it graduated into a much heavier flow. I became bedridden and was worried about the amount of blood I was losing. And then, one night I awoke to find that I was hemorrhaging!

I made an emergency call to my doctor and ended up in the hospital with an extremely low hemoglobin count. I needed a massive blood transfusion. I learned that some women experience severe bleeding during the onset of their menopause. My male gynecologist was far from being detached and unsympathetic. He was very concerned and wanted to avoid the possibility of another transfusion. We had a long discussion in which he explained that I had an important decision to face. He said that I had two options. At this point, I made a decision that marked a radical departure from what almost every American woman before me had experienced. Allow me to explain.

I had the option of having a hysterectomy, which would stop the severe bleeding by removing my uterus but would spare my ovaries, or I could try a new procedure that had only been done on thirteen women in the world to date. Whoa! He candidly told me that he hated to see me have the hysterectomy, because one of the side effects was rapid premature aging. Often, the skin of the face and body grows dry and wrinkled soon after the removal of the uterus.

The other option was a revolutionary method of uterine ablation — called the "roller ball" treatment. This procedure, developed by Dr. Duane Townsend, at the time a uterine oncologist at Cedars-Sinai Medical Center, involved the use of a laser tool the size and shape of a ballpoint pen. The instrument would be introduced vaginally and inserted into the uterus. The lining of the uterus would be burned or singed, eradicating the blood vessels that carry the menstrual blood. This new method offered all the benefits of a hysterectomy, but since I'd still retain my uterus as well as my ovaries, there would be no accelerated aging. It was the procedure that provided the least radical approach. Later, the uterus could be removed if necessary, but that might never be required. I couldn't keep from wondering how a man who had prostate problems would react if his doctor recommended having his entire prostate removed.

I decided to go with the new procedure. I was ready to be a guinea pig, because all the other surgeries of this type had proved successful, plus it seemed like an ingenious approach to a very complicated problem. I traveled to Sacramento, where Dr. Townsend was performing this special surgery; since he had invented the method and had done the other surgeries, I chose to have him do it. During the surgery, my cervix had to be dilated, which brought on painful cramps like childbirth. When it was all over, I was happy with my decision and grateful for the suggestion in the first place. I felt blessed to reap the benefit of this forward-reaching medical breakthrough. I'm sure that today many more woman are undergoing this kind of procedure, instead of what now seems almost barbaric . . . the removal of the entire uterus at the onset of menopause.

The truth is that all the organs of the body have functions that interact with the rest of the internal system. As women, we should be very cautious, if given the choice, about removing pieces of ourselves, particularly the sexual organs that govern and generate important hormones. It was previously thought that female reproductive organs were "dispensable" after childbearing age. Now we know that our reproductive organs produce hormones, particularly estrogen, progesterone, and to a lesser degree testosterone, and that these are essential for our quality of life. Besides reproduction, these hormones are responsible for so many physical and mental aspects of our well-being. Now, I am not, of course, an M.D. and certainly don't intend to make medical recommendations, but I do want to cover the various hormone-replacement therapies and other related treatments that worked and didn't work for me. Indeed, I went through a wide range of experimentation before my system finally leveled out.

Hormone-Replacement Therapy

Some women don't need hormonal support . . . I, however, am among those who do. Once I survived "the change," I emerged on the other side of the looking glass feeling sadly depleted. The loss of energy and a slump in my morale left me dragging. I needed help. Like millions of my sisters around the world, I began a program of hormone-replacement therapy, or HRT.

Talk about Alice in Wonderland! What a menagerie of hormonal options, tablets, potions, creams, gels, and patches there are to choose from! It's rather like shopping for shoes; you feel compelled to try them all on until you find the perfect fit. But it's a very tricky proposition, because no two women are alike. That's where networking kicks in, and it can help. You can learn from the experience of your girlfriends and the women in your family and they from you; otherwise, during this trial-and-error phase, driven by the need to find relief from your symptoms, you're likely to feel like a guinea pig testing dozens of different formulas and preparations.

It's truly remarkable that women's health issues seem to have dragged behind and not kept pace with technological advances in so many other medical fields. But the demands of boomers for better and safer solutions to treat "the change" have prompted a wave of viable options for us to choose from. The newest approach is based on *bio-identical hormones* and a more sophisticated understanding of what damage can be caused in the female body by the use of *unopposed estrogen*. Many women, in the hope of rejuvenation through HRT, have caused themselves a lot of grief and have even needed surgical procedures to undo the damage. However, millions have benefited from hormone replacement when it's balanced effectively and customized to their individual body chemistry.

Estrogen

The female body self-generates three kinds of estrogen: estrone, estradiol, and estriol. Estrone is usually produced and stored in the fatty areas of the body, such as the hips, thighs, and breasts, and is the form most prescribed. Estradiol is the second most commonly prescribed form of estrogen and has many of the same qualities as estrone. Estriol is another, less-aggressive choice and is thought to possess a preventive quality in regard to cancer. Today's women usually find estriol to be their preferred solution, because it is reputed to be better for women with increased concerns about breast cancer. All forms of estrogen come in a wide range of applications including patches that adhere to the skin, tablets taken orally or sublingually (under the tongue), and creams applied to the skin. Some formulas are synthetic versions of the natural hormones produced by the body; but as mentioned before, the ideal form of these estrogens is a bio-identical formula. Bio-identical hormones are created in a laboratory by altering compounds derived from naturally occurring plant products.

The popularity of HRT using estrogen stems from its reported positive effects in decreasing the risk of heart disease, osteoporosis, and hot flashes. It also boosts HDL (the good cholesterol), prevents vaginal thinning and dryness, and is very beneficial to the skin, dramatically improving its tone and retarding the appearances of wrinkles. No wonder it is so widely used! It is important to emphasize that "unopposed" estrogen — meaning estrogen taken alone over time — can stimulate the growth of uterine fibroids, cause thickening of the uterine lining, and even promote the growth of cancer cells. The cancer usually appears first in the uterus or various other female organs such as the breasts and ovaries but often spreads to other organs of the body. For this reason, understandably, estrogen therapy has been the subject of much controversy and negative publicity as medical reports on these effects are released.

The old-fashioned, almost automatic prescription for menopausal symptoms for my mother's generation was Premarin. Premarin is a form of estrogen in a tablet, which is concocted from a collection of more than twenty different equine estrogens mostly made from the urine of pregnant mares.[1] Personally, I couldn't care less what it's made from, but this fact makes many people cringe. And yet, millions of women have benefited from taking it in tandem with a form of progesterone known as Provera. Conventional wisdom, supported by the medical community, says that estrogen must *always* be taken with progesterone to prevent estrogen dominance. Taken together, these two hormones still remain a mainstay for many women today. Nonetheless, this popular dynamic duo did not turn out to be the answer for me. The Premarin was not the problem, but Provera did not agree with my body chemistry. So I was forced to seek out other solutions.

In a situation like this, what every woman needs first and foremost is a qualified and reputable gynecologist who specializes and has ample experience in menopausal treatments. Thank God women over the past two decades have realized that a cookie-cutter remedy for "the change" is outdated. Women are now rightfully demanding more individualized care and relying on their "gynos" to customize their treatment. Any doctor worth his or her salt will order *a complete blood and salivary profile to assess your individual hormone imbalances*, before deciding on a program of therapy. I like the physicians who are familiar with herbal and natural remedies rather than those who are too quick to give conventional allopathic medication for every menopause malady. Yet, if that's what you need, there is nothing wrong with taking it. And then, of course, it's essential to follow up with testing for any side effects, to track how your body is responding and to determine whether you need to continue taking these supplements or prescriptions and for how long.

Clearly, I'm not qualified to make medical recommendations, but I do want to cover the various treatments that worked and didn't work for me. Far from the slam dunk I would have preferred, I waded through a wide range of experiments before my system finally leveled out. But

---

[1]As described by Christiane Northrup, M.D., in her wonderful book *Women's Bodies, Women's Wisdom*.

then again, I've always been eager to learn about new treatments and how to maximize my health. It seems to come naturally to me, and I would encourage every woman to listen to her doctor's advice but also to stay well informed so she can be her own health-care advocate. Thank God for the doctors and their care; but we also have a responsibility to our own bodies and often can help our caregivers by asking questions and informing them about what is going on with us. I see this as a collaborative relationship.

As I've experienced it, one's body chemistry seems to change every five to seven years. Treatments and practices that once worked may very well need to be changed or updated. You may have to come up with a whole new recipe or hormonal cocktail to fit the new cycle you are currently in. When I first started taking estrogen, it seemed very effective at the outset for boosting my energy and keeping me on an even keel. But before long—because of the cumulative effects of HRT—I could see that I was retaining water. Though my face was free of wrinkles, it looked much fuller than before, and my dress size ballooned, until soon I couldn't zip up my favorite clothes.

Yikes! Naturally, I went on a diet and jacked up my cardio, but things only improved slightly. Besides, every time I took progesterone, it seemed to bring me down, and no one seemed able to explain to me why. It was time to find a better answer, because I wasn't satisfied with the side effects of either the estrogen or the progesterone. Then, sure enough, I became a lab rat for all manner of cream formulas, which resulted in feeling "up" one minute and like a limp rag the next. This wasn't fun, and it was very expensive. While searching for a solution to my hormone imbalance, I was making a handful of compounding pharmacies (pharmacies that customize hormone formulas) very rich!

The problem with hormone therapy is that the individual dosage and the exact ratio between progesterone and estrogen are crucial; and sometimes, if it's just a fraction of a microgram off, it doesn't work. As my first couple of years of experimentation wore on, I began to use transdermal patches of estrogen. I was taking .05 milligrams of estrogen, delivered through the skin, and I could tell that my symptoms were easing up. But there was a catch. Even though the patches bypass the liver, which is a plus, they also release a higher dose of hormones than those taken orally. And with my highly sensitive chemistry, this caused water retention and weight gain, *too*. I had to accept that I would probably never be a size 4 again.

When I was on Broadway in the '90s, the dancing and rehearsing for six to eight hours a day would eat up the estrogen and I'd feel faint and weak. Even so, I pressed on knowing that a whole company of people were depending on me. Whereas in premenopause there had been a cushion of reserve that allowed me to go with the flow, I now felt I was on shaky ground. Each situation seemed to require a different dosage. Somehow I managed to muddle through for the run of the play, but it was far from ideal.

Eventually, I found myself in the office of a doctor who actually prescribed almost double the amount of estrogen that I'd been taking. That proved to be a serious mistake and forced me to undergo another surgical procedure to remove the fibroids and polyps that had grown as a result of this folly. Yes, the high doses of estrogen were responsible. Fortunately, none of the tissue was cancerous. Hallelujah! After that, I weaned myself off hormones completely . . . but it took eighteen months to accomplish that. I've been off hormone-replacement therapy ever since.

When exploring HRT for the first time, I wasn't prepared for the powerful effects they could have, not just on the female organs, but on my whole mental and emotional state. I had tried birth control pills when I was younger, the kind in those little dial-pack disks, but they made me nauseous, so I never climbed aboard the birth-control wagon. I didn't know anyone who did! I think we children of the Eisenhower era just sensed when we were ovulating and adjusted accordingly.

Not to digress, but I've always wondered why women's cancers have grown to such epidemic proportions since the '50s. Legions of women have been on the Pill since then, and with each new decade, girls are becoming sexually active earlier and earlier. By the time they get older, they have already saturated their system with hormones that consistently interfere with their reproductive cycles to such a degree that it would seem likely such doses could have detrimental effects. As a matter of fact, the National Cancer Institute cites at least one established link between the Pill and increased incidences of liver cancer in women. I find it helpful that the FDA and surgeon general require a list of side effects and warnings on the literature accompanying all ingested contraceptives— as they do on cigarettes. Personally, I think there's a lot to be said for women becoming more sensitive to their own menstrual cycles and taking charge of their reproductive health in a responsible way.

The Adrenal Glands

Another symptom of menopause is low adrenal function, which can lead to a loss of energy and the onslaught of depression. The adrenal glands are mood-elevating twins situated just on top of the kidneys. They are responsible for the ability to approach each day with vigor, a clear mind, and a positive attitude. So when the adrenals break down, we feel like the rug has been pulled out from under us.

They are also our natural emergency support system. When the adrenal twins are called into action, due to fear, anxiety or stress, or even excitement in the positive sense, they come to the rescue by producing adrenaline, cortisol, and DHEA. The proper ratio between your level of DHEA and cortisol contributes greatly to a strong, healthy life. However, during menopause, when hormones are reduced, this balance is often thrown out of whack. Thus, women who suffer from low or depleted adrenals often have more difficulty during menopause.

I happen to be a woman who suffers from low adrenal function, which has sometimes aggravated my menopausal symptoms. I'm a health and exercise enthusiast, but there were times when, even with the best of intentions, I could not get through a workout. So I needed to investigate the cause of my diminishing stamina. It's never easy, but if you understand that you're not alone in this quest, it boosts your morale and also helps you stay more proactive.

I discovered that my adrenals were exhausted, as the result of two factors. One was the lack of sufficient nutritional support, and the other was my lifestyle. I'll discuss nutritional support and diet in the next chapter, but I'd like to make it clear that each woman must customize her diet to support the activities she has chosen to participate in. You wouldn't expect a car to run without fuel and oil; nor can you expect your poor adrenals to function without sufficient protein in your diet. The other factor is psychological stress, which is related to what kind of thoughts, words and actions you allow yourself to indulge in.

For example, low adrenals are often the result of an overambitious schedule or too much unchecked—either positive or negative—emotional involvement in your current activities. The adrenal twins, like Thelma and Louise, can become way too emotionally charged and get caught up in a chain of foolish reactions. The same syndrome could be true of you. Allowing worry and anxiety to run rampant over rational thinking can severely impact your life choices and play havoc with your adrenals. And so it's very important when you're feeling low to reexamine your current reactions to people and situations surrounding your daily activities. You cannot change how others behave, but you *are* in control of your own thoughts and responses. On another note, there are also times when we simply try too hard, forcing ourselves beyond our limits and thereby taxing our adrenals. It's okay to lighten up on your workload and rest when you feel tired or take some time off for recreation. A change of perspective can truly help your adrenals recover. Why not cut yourself some slack and take a break from that ambitious ego?

It's important to identify negative thoughts: your hates and dislikes, your fears, angers, and resentments, which cause you to become emotionally charged. Once you invite such loaded thoughts *in* and harbor them, in the corners of your mind, they're like a time bomb waiting to go off, making it almost impossible to override your explosive impulses. Even though you may have mastered the art of appearing very poised and in control, a calm exterior will not defuse the toxic effect such emotions will have on your poor adrenals.

Emotional impulses become even more heightened during menopause, and you may have noticed some of the following symptoms:

- ✓ Fatigue and exhaustion
- ✓ Chronic insomnia
- ✓ Dependence on caffeine upon arising and nearly nonstop throughout the day
- ✓ A tendency to rehash situations and to worry constantly
- ✓ Insufficient nutrition, probably caused by a decrease in your ability to absorb nutrients due to stress
- ✓ Deep-seated anger, resentment, fear, depression, and guilt. Chronic feelings hovering just beneath the surface. These can be either about past or present concerns. Such emotions can be caused or even aggravated by low adrenals.
- ✓ Certain allergies
- ✓ Hypoglycemia

If you can identify the symptoms listed above as your own, then perhaps you should explore your adrenal, cortisol, and DHEA levels. *A salivary test is the most accurate method of doing so.* According to the renowned doctor and author John R. Lee, the foremost authority on natural progesterone, *blood tests often do not accurately show these levels.*

There are other phenomena that can cause added stress for the adrenal-challenged woman, including recovery from illness, surgery, or trauma, either mental or physical; radical change of occupation; change of climate; too much or too little exposure to the sun; too much humidity; traveling and time zone changes, which can disrupt sleep cycles and digestive patterns; and moving out of your home. It's quite possible that during such times you could use some help to support your adrenal system while it copes with unusual and trying circumstances.

Progesterone

Enter the opposing hormone called progesterone. Most often it is used together with some form of estrogen. However, there is a growing school of thought, led by Dr. Lee, that maintains that, because progesterone is a precursor of estrogen, the proper dose can stimulate the production of estrogen at a nondominant level. When, as I described earlier in this chapter, progesterone is used as a partner with estrogen, the dosage needs to be balanced precisely to avoid stimulating the estrogen receptors in the uterus and breasts. Moreover, it has also been proved through clinical research that many women prefer to use progesterone on its own and have achieved very good results.

The popularity of progesterone therapy has grown over the past decade or so. It is available in both tablet and cream form. The recommended approach is to take a daily bioidentical progesterone supplement alone in cream form.

I've personally become very interested in progesterone because it is reputed to offer better support to the adrenal glands and provide a balanced level of DHEA (a precursor for testosterone) and cortisol. Even in my postmenopausal years, I am looking for a way to stimulate my adrenal glands without the use of estrogen, which is, as I've stated, problematic for me. In the final analysis, it all depends on the individual user, her reaction to progesterone and her specific needs—every woman should have her progesterone levels tested through a salivary panel before a supplemental program is prescribed. It's a path definitely worth discussing with your qualified physician.

Testosterone

If you are using an effective progesterone supplement, then you should already have your testosterone covered. However, others on estrogen and progesterone supplements may still feel under par in certain areas. In that case, these women may want to ask their doctor about testing their level of testosterone, for example, in case of low sexual desire. Testosterone is usually taken in very low dosages, such as 1 or 2 milligrams every other day and sometimes in a topical cream form. Too much of it can result in unwanted facial hair and, occasionally, overly aggressive behavior. Consult a qualified physician who is knowledgeable about HRT.

Nutritional Supplements

There is a plethora of excellent vitamin and herbal supplements that are very useful in treating hot flashes, brain fog, circulation problems, low adrenals, joint pain, and osteoporosis, many of which are problems associated with menopause and aging.

An extensive list of the nutritional supplements that I personally take are listed on page 94 of chapter 7. Please check it out.

Human Growth Hormone, aka HGH

This is a highly controversial subject. Human growth hormone is one of the many hormones produced by the body, like estrogen, progesterone, and testosterone, all of which are triggered by the pituitary gland. HGH is at its highest level in childhood and adolescence, when it facilitates intensified growth, as the name suggests. It decreases with age and menopause, just like other hormones. The replacement of HGH is purported to have very broad-reaching anti-aging benefits for men and women alike. Some books and medical journals report that HGH *may* have some of the following benefits: the restoration of muscle mass, a decrease in body fat, reduction of wrinkles by thickening the skin, reversing hair loss and restoring hair color, increasing energy and sexual function, improving the cholesterol profile, improving vision and memory, elevating mood, and improving sleep. It is also said to increase stamina and support the liver, pancreas, heart, and other organs. Sounds like a dream come true! Unfortunately, HGH doesn't always live up to the hype.

I've had only one experience with taking this hormone, during the shooting of *American Family*, a television series I was working on several years ago. The hours were grueling on this weekly series, and my gynecologist at the time suggested that I take very low doses of injectable HGH, which I administered to myself with an insulin needle each morning when I got up. I was initially worried about mild side effects, because it is a steroid; you may recall that certain weightlifters who have taken steroids display prominent foreheads and exaggerated brow lines. They have the look of Neanderthal man. No woman would want this to happen.

I can't say that HGH gave me any discernible boost or rush of energy or any pronounced change in my skin or hair, but it did help my stamina and mental alertness for several months, despite the grueling hours. It also seemed to buffer the drag on my nerves that came with the pressure of learning and performing new dialogue every day. Nonetheless, I discontinued taking HGH after filming ended. I saw no need for the added support in my daily life and knew from experience with hormone replacement therapy that the cumulative effects of *any* hormone supplement can result in undesirable consequences. Proceed with caution!

Eight years later, at a time when I felt consistently exhausted and under par, I asked my gynecologist to prescribe HGH for me. However, this time the solution was from a different lab, with a different brand name. After only ten days on these injections, I noticed that I was looking "puffy" in photographs, and I discontinued use immediately. So, when exploring this area, pay very close attention to every aspect of your reaction to HGH, making sure to have follow-up blood tests, which any reputable physician should insist on. In my opinion, men who take HGH seem to be less sensitive than women to such factors as thickening of the skin and exaggerated muscle mass. We, on the other hand, should be more careful. I always recall that the famous and beloved Olympic champion, Florence Griffith-Joyner, who some speculate died a premature death precipitated by her use of steroids.

FIVE

Preventive Aging

WHAT CAN BE DONE TO MAKE THE EN-
croaching years feel and look better? In our new age, with all its prom-
ising resources aimed at preventive aging, this is certainly an area of
interest for all men and women, including those in their twenties and
thirties. It's never too early to devote time and energy to protecting and
maintaining our health and appearance. Aging well depends on how old
you are when you finally decide to take "preventive" action.

If you're in your forties, then you've hit the smokin' high point of
your prime . . . and you'll need to make the most of it to ensure your
longevity and maintain a youthful appearance. Plus, you've still got all
those sexy hormones and should be feeling pretty frisky. You know in
your heart that you've still got what it takes to get out there and kick
it. So go ahead and own it!

Your forties is the time when you may also be hoping to avoid the
perils of "the change." I can only tell you that the onset of menopause
is very different for each woman. I have always found that most symptoms in the female cycle, including the fluctuations of your menstrual
hormones and endocrine system, are very susceptible to stress levels,
both emotional and physical. It's also my theory that emotional patterns
of stress, or driving yourself hard physically, can, over time, etch a blue-

print on your monthly cycles. This can later affect how menopause unfolds in your life. If you take hormones for various contraceptive or regulating reasons, this too could affect menopause and your risk of reproductive cancers. Finally, premature menopause, as I understand it, can sometimes be caused by thinning of the uterine lining from having multiple D&C procedures or other surgical work done on the reproductive organs, or any other practice that alters your hormones or cycles.

However, it's hard to predict how menopause will affect you and when it will come. Some are fortunate and have a smooth ride, and so much depends on inherited genes and lifestyle. I think consulting a knowledgeable gynecologist is the best way to regulate the shifting of estrogen and progesterone levels during the perimenopausal phase. A doctor must monitor these changes as they come, and only a professional — or perhaps a female relative — can be insightful enough to answer the myriad questions applicable to you. Even so, I see menopause and its side effects as a very inexact and variable area of medical science, though women tend to feel that there *should* be a one-size-fits-all answer. There isn't one, as far as I know.

Once you're fifty or older, you've acquired a much clearer perspective on life, which allows you to look backward and make assessments; but also to glance forward with a better sense of self and what your priorities are for the future.

Menopause can feel like a downward slide. I felt that I'd crossed the line where time was no longer on my side. I figured that all my efforts to maintain my health and appearance would reap diminishing returns. What a bummer! I started to feel depressed by the prospect of losing the age game. What brought me out of the doldrums was the thought of how resilient my mother had always been. She was the original iron butterfly . . . *sooo* feminine in manner, but like Smokin' Joe Frazier when it came to figuratively taking a punch. You just couldn't keep her down. I later found myself following her example, prodding myself to forge ahead in spite of discouraging odds; and it has served me well into my fifties and beyond.

We all have an inner voice, call it intuition, that lets us know exactly how old or young we truly are and how we feel about it. As you round each year, it becomes clearer that real insight comes from that voice within. Listen to it and ignore the outside judgments and influences. It's up to you to recognize precisely who you are and what you want out of life. Don't be persuaded otherwise by a number. Just focus in on your own strengths and set your sights on achieving your goals.

Women are great at planning ahead, and you have the perfect chance all through your forties, fifties, and beyond to make a liar out of the calendar and probably shave a decade off your chronological age! Preventive aging is similar to *preventive medicine* and describes what I consider the wisest philosophy of aging gracefully. If you get busy, you can actually *prevent, retard, or delay the aging process . . . or even reverse it*. On the other hand, if you've neglected yourself and are getting alarmed that your age is showing and accelerating—or if you've suffered through a debilitating illness, injury, or depression—you'll need to slow down or stall the aging process. But don't despair; regardless of your age, the body is still very resilient and responsive to anti-aging techniques. I can testify that you'll likely be able to *retard* and *reverse* some of the visible signs of aging. But if you're like me, you'll probably prefer to get an earlier start and deal with *prevention* rather than *reversal*. Prevention has better odds.

Think of aging gracefully as a game. We might as well make up our minds to play it, or just bow out and be spectators. There's nothing wrong with the latter. It's a valid choice, if you don't mind hardening of the arteries, osteoporosis, arthritis, and senility. In other words, sitting around doing nothing is far from the best option. Just as you maintain your home, your car, your garden, etc., you should look after your greatest gift . . . your body. Besides, fitness and beauty go hand in hand. So now is the time to start making an ongoing commitment to preventive techniques. I'm not talking about liposuction . . . no, I'm referring to letting the miracle of your body work for you. Of course, it's going to take some discipline and effort. But it's undoubtedly worth it.

Miracle of the Body

Consider the natural healing power of the human body, and imagine the potential we can unleash if we nurture that power and direct it in a positive, healthy way. It's phenomenal! I love the axiom "The body is the temple of the spirit." So true! We're given this spectacular anatomy, this exceptional organism in which to house our soul . . . in which to live our life. I, for one, have come to feel an obligation to look after it. It deserves our respect and attention. If we treat it like the treasure it is, it will serve us incredibly well in return. Whatever investment you put into your body and mind is bound to gather interest like money in the bank and pay you back a hundredfold.

My body is the shape I live in
and it shapes the way I live. — R.W.

It doesn't matter whether you walk, jog, bicycle, swim, play tennis, golf, dance, jump rope, lift weights, or do Pilates; the important thing is that you find a discipline that keeps you physically active on a regular basis, and schedule it for a certain time each day. Your longevity, quality of life, and youthfulness depend on it.

You'll need to develop a comfort level within whatever activity you choose. You know as well as I do that in situations like this, we often start one thing and then stop, try something else, and so on. Think of it as a quest. Choosing an exercise program or physical pursuit for the first time is like finding a new best friend. This "fitness friend" is going to sustain you for years to come. If you already have something that has worked for you, pick up where you left off. All of us fall off the wagon and get lazy, only to regret it.

I have to admit that I floundered around for quite a while before settling on something that offered me the results and experience I craved. There was a lot of trial and error, until I literally stumbled upon a method that worked for me, one that fit my needs, both physically and mentally. So if at first you don't succeed, don't give up. I'm not suggesting that you follow my exact routine. We're clearly not all the same. I merely offer my experience to inspire you to get out there and assemble your own customized preventive program.

Here is a checklist of my essential requirements for age prevention and physical fitness.

Cardio training Cardiovascular conditioning is vitally important for the heart and lungs. One of my mentors used to say that the marriage between the heart and lungs was a difficult mating game. They have to be persuaded to cooperate with each other by regular walking, climbing, jumping rope, using an elliptical machine or treadmill, or practicing any number of sports. It's remarkable how you can chase your aches and pains away with movement. Cardio activity also burns calories, which is important for weight control if you want to drop pounds. It also builds stamina, and "breaking a sweat" helps to cleanse the body of impurities. You'll find that you look forward to this activity, because it acts as a mood elevator through endorphins.

. Be sure to drink water following this type of exercise to rehydrate your body. Your daily water consumption should be the equivalent of two 1.5 liter bottles per day, just over one and a half quarts. Water intake also helps to curb your appetite.

Strength training You can build strength using weights or working the machine circuit at a gym, but resistance training such as Pilates is also especially effective for women. As you get older, weight or resistance training to contract and activate the muscles is super important to ward off osteoporosis. Women in particular tend to lose muscle mass with age, so you need to keep your muscles active and strong, because weakening muscles put added strain on the joints, especially your hips and knees. So I incorporate weight training into my regular routine three times a week. You'll need to engage each week in a total workout, divided between the upper and lower body. This should include abdominals or *core training*, which is addressed beautifully by the Pilates method, and the larger muscle groups of the back, shoulders, and *latissimi dorsi*, or "lats." If you want to sculpt and tone your upper arms, which is a common concern, you can use free weights to shape the biceps and triceps.

The larger muscle groups of the lower body, like the "glutes," abs, and thighs, need regular maintenance. There are numerous videos that target these areas. For your buns, try squats with a five-pound weight in each hand. Leg lifts with ankle weights usually work well. Also try lunges. However, I recommend that you have a qualified trainer outline a specific program for you. Any weight-bearing exercise needs to be carefully performed to be effective and injury free.

Flexibility training   This type of exercise is wonderful for preventing or reducing joint pain and stiffness despite arthritis and for increasing or maintaining range of movement. It also aids the flow of synovial fluid. Synovial fluid is the indispensable lubricating fluid present in most of our joints. It is the "juice" that enables the two separate bones that intersect to move freely where they come together. Your knee for example is designed with cartilage that cushions the ends of the bones, but the synovial fluid is the "oil" that allows the whole mechanism to operate smoothly without discomfort. Joint movement and flexibility training help circulate synovial fluid through the joint and nourish the cartilage with oxygen, promoting healthy joint tissue. As we age, the goal is to combat arthritis and be very respectful of the joints. We have to be more selective about what surfaces we stand and work on, and what kind of shoes we wear. There are, of course, many choices of athletic footwear, but be careful about enough toe room and comfort for walking and exercise. Low impact and careful, gradual movement, as in yoga and Pilates, are best for avoiding injury and accommodating an existing condition like arthritis or joint inflammation. Easy does it . . . slow and steady is really the surest way to get positive results.

Relaxation and stress relief   Relaxation rids the body and mind of stress. It is commonly known that mental and emotional stress in particular have adverse effects on every single organ of the body, including the brain, impairing our judgment and causing anxiety. We all need a change of pace, a vacation, the solace and support of friends and family and just plain ol' downtime, like a good book or a good night's sleep. In addition, by midlife many of our stress-related complaints have become chronic, so we need to regularly still the mind and the body through reliable methods. I'm speaking of meditation, breathing techniques, and yoga postures that induce a relaxed state. The stress level fallout from the computer age is off the hook. Because of this constant assault on our senses, what might have once been optional is now vital to our sanity and well-being.

There seems to be a cacophony of noise, conflicting messages, and interference rattling around in our heads, making it harder and harder to distinguish between the heart and core of a matter and the constant static that impedes our natural mental process. It's an age of too much information (TMI). Uninvited interruptions and superfluous racket threaten to drown out sanity and clear thinking. They also cause a disconnect with the true inner self. I believe it was my unconscious need to open my heart and reconnect to my inner voice that led me to yoga.

Yoga by Way of Vegas

How did I arrive at the right choice of method in my search? It happened almost by accident. Strangely enough it was in Las Vegas, of all places! Talk about superfluous racket . . . *ka-ching!* It was the mid '70s and I was headlining for the first time at the International Hilton. This was Elvis turf, and I got to stay in the lavish Elvis Presley Penthouse with breathtaking views of the Strip below. I was even more blown away when I got word that following my final show, I would meet Elvis himself, for the second time in my life.

It had been ten years or more since I'd appeared — as an unknown — in the Elvis movie *Roustabout*. It was my first Hollywood movie (blink and you'll miss me), so I doubted "El" would remember me.

Anyway, on closing night, BJ Ward, my lead backup singer, stopped by my dressing room before the show to go over some vocals and found me stressing over leg raises with Velcro ankle weights. She could see by my face how much I hated it.

"Hey Rocky, why don't you try yoga?" she suggested. I politely declined. This was back in the '70s, and like a lot of people back then, I had a built-in resistance to yoga. Was it a sect? Was there a swami? Was it voodoo? It sounded much too weird, and besides, I was allergic to incense. It made me sneeze.

Since then I've come to understand that my girlfriend had just opened the door to a life-changing experience . . . one that I practice religiously to this day. Some of you may recall that I wrote a bestselling book on the subject, circa 1983, entitled *Raquel: Total Beauty and Fitness*, which was miles ahead of its time. Fortunately, these days we can find a yoga studio on every street corner. Back in the day it was pretty rare.

I eventually took BJ's advice and embraced yoga, which doubled my energy, increased my muscle tone and flexibility, and banished my emotional stress levels. It's not hard to understand why I became a devotee. The icing on the cake was that yoga had a rejuvenating effect on my face and body . . . Hel-lo! I was sold. And to think I stumbled upon something so esoteric in the raucous gambling capital of the world! Plus, I got to see Elvis again, up close and personal. And he did remember me!

Achieving Your Goals Inside and Out

I chose yoga as my anti-aging method because I discovered that it incorporates almost all the key elements I listed above: cardio, flexibility, strength training, and stress relief. More importantly, whether it's Garbo or Swanson, Madonna or Gwyneth Paltrow, the rejuvenating effects of yoga are evident. In addition, this renowned Eastern discipline is designed to stimulate the endocrine glands, which govern the entire hormonal system. I'll describe this in more detail shortly.

Yoga also encompasses two essential yet opposing factors, which constantly interact and cannot be divided. It's impossible to address one without affecting the other. That's the genius of the way we are created. I'm speaking of the *mind-body connection*, which is now an official course of scientific study at Harvard Medical School. Together, the mind and the body, when working in harmony, can radically impact those desirable inner (character) and outer (physical) traits that grace a woman with timeless appeal. Without focusing on both mind and body, you will not achieve the best result from your preventive aging routine. Put simply, you have to cultivate a *healthy mind (attitude) in a healthy body and vice versa*.

The Endocrine System

There are two main reasons why yoga is universally effective as an anti-aging tool. First, a comprehensive yoga practice affects the entire endocrine system by methodically stimulating each and every one of the hormonal glands and causing them to function at optimum efficiency — at any age. This is not something that I've heard identified very often. But when I started this practice, I became keenly aware of the rejuvenating benefits of yoga: not just the way it shaped my body, but especially the effect it had on my skin and complexion. The endocrine glands I'm referring to include: the *pineal, pituitary, thyroid, parathyroid,* and *adrenals*. These major glands govern energy levels, mental clarity, and muscle tone as well as the quality, color, and overall appearance of your skin. They also positively affect your mental state and sleep patterns, among other functions.

The reason yoga has a positive impact on the hormonal system is that many of the postures direct the blood flow toward the head, where the pituitary and pineal glands are located. Think of it . . . how many times a day is your head in a position lower than your heart? Almost never. But in yoga practice, it happens frequently by design. This is important because circulation to the pineal and pituitary glands is increased and these glands govern the rest of the endocrine network. Obviously, you can't go around upside down, and it's not necessary, because a regular yoga routine will suffice.

One of yoga's most famous postures is the *headstand*, but there are several easier options as well. I've managed to accomplish the same benefits with *semi-inverted yoga poses*, which don't put so much pressure on the neck. These are done while kneeling or standing upright and bending forward slowly toward the floor from the hips. Almost any yoga book has a variety of such poses to choose from, and most can be performed by people of all ages. You'll see the visible effects on your skin and hair very quickly with regular practice. However, done isolated on their own as a trick, instead of as part of a series, these positions are much less effective. It's like making a soufflé . . . every single ingredient and detail is essential to the final creation.

The Central Nervous System

The second but equally important benefit of yoga is that it *conditions and realigns the spine*, which houses the all-important *central nervous system*. Generally speaking, if you have a healthy spine, you have a healthy body and life. The snakelike structure of the spine is made up of twenty-six movable parts called vertebrae. It's brilliant! Individual nerves extend out through the extremities like tentacles and are traceable back to the spine as the hub, like Grand Central Station. It's very useful to fully understand how the life energy supplied by each spinal nerve is fed through the system. The nervous system tracks all the byways throughout the body. It's an amazing work of art. Ancient yoga positions have been designed to correspond to and stimulate all the vital organs, glands, and tissues of the body.

Curative Effects of Circulation

It has been said that, generally speaking, all illness is the result of a lack of circulation, leading to congestion of the arteries, heart, lungs, and lymphatic system, and even the cellular composition of the body. It's also essential to the healing process. When you're feeling poorly, or even when you're recovering from an injury, the sooner you start moving and get your circulation flowing again, the sooner you'll be on the road to recovery. The yoga technique for improving circulation is quite unique. Allow me to explain. The word *yoga* is Sanskrit for union, so the rule is that whatever move you execute must be counterbalanced by doing the opposite movement. In other words, when you bend forward, then you must also bend backward to balance the spine. When you bend to the right, follow through by bending to the left. It is a system of balance designed to increase circulation, without the physical impact of other methods. The velocity of the blood flow increases when the body radically changes direction from head to toe, causing this life-giving fluid to course through the veins of the torso from stem to stern. For example: with arms raised high over head, by bending down slowly from the hips gradually in an arc-like manner to touch the feet and then by reversing the process, rising slowly back up to the starting position, you can activate a stream of vital blood flowing throughout the total system. It's the opposite of shaking yourself up in a violent way, like a bottle of ketchup. Have you ever noticed that a river *runs* and the sea is never absolutely still? Stagnant water grows all kinds of scum, bacteria, and disease. And so it goes with our bodies. Systematic stirring of the blood flow, directing it to nourish every single organ, ensures healing and rejuvenation.

The trunk of the body also needs to be tuned up in a comprehensive manner, to assist the adrenal glands and spine to operate at optimum efficiency. With improved circulation, your digestion, colon, and kidney function, as well as the pancreas, liver, and spleen are all nourished and conditioned so they can do their job of detoxifying and cleansing the body.

We hear a lot about "detoxing," which is one of the benefits of good circulation. This should remind us that the care and maintenance of our "one and only" body is a sacred duty; even more important than changing the oil in your car or cleaning your house and not leaving any dirty dishes in the sink. So if you're interested in looking and feeling younger, aim to make your daily practice as automatic as brushing your teeth.

SIX

Destination Yoga

LET ME PREFACE EVERYTHING BY CLARIFYING that *Hatha* yoga, the kind I practice, is not *passive* meditation. It isn't about *om-m-ing* out. Hatha yoga is a form of exercise—I prefer to call it a discipline—that originated in India as a *preparation for meditation.* Once you become more accomplished in practicing yoga, the process often develops naturally into a form of *active* meditation. In other words, yoga teaches you how to maintain relaxed concentration and movement simultaneously. Why is this necessary? Because most Westerners cannot just plop down and meditate or sit still for even five minutes without fidgeting restlessly, unable to release their minds from the grip of daily strife. I say this because I tried my hand at transcendental meditation back in the '60s, only to find that repeating my assigned mantra over and over again, like a chant, made me strangely anxious and surprisingly hostile! I doubt that this happens to everyone, but the experience taught me that I was really not *ready* for meditation . . . I needed to clear up some anxiety issues first. Not so unexpected, given the years I'd spent carrying around the uncomfortable mantle of sex symbol while caught in the glare of the public eye. My gal pal, BJ, had been right. Boy, did I need yoga.

Rejuvenating Benefits

The anti-aging benefits of yoga break down into five key categories:

1. First, you'll notice a decided improvement in the appearance of both your face and body. Your body will look more sculpted and toned and you'll simply love the skin you're in.
2. Also, your spine, nervous system and entire skeletal structure, along with your posture, should improve.
3. Joint flexibility, as well as range of motion, will increase, making you more agile and giving you freedom of movement with less discomfort. Thus, physical activity will become easier, as though you were years younger.
4. The health and function of all your internal organs should improve, especially those age-defying glands, which govern the production of hormones.
5. You will become aware of those inherent inner qualities or character virtues that automatically start to develop as part of your practice.

The beauty of yoga is that your character tends to improve simultaneously as you meet your physical goals. This is more proof that the *mind-body connection* is potent and inescapable. Many desirable character virtues are achieved as a direct result of the self-correction you experience while utilizing an authentic yoga method.

Among these character virtues are:

✓ Patience = Serenity
✓ Concentration = Focus
✓ Balance = Equilibrium
✓ Flexibility = Versatility

✓ Determination = Discipline
✓ Faith = Confidence
✓ Coordination = Agility

As you examine the list above, it should become evident how such virtues can enable you to reshape your life and pursue your personal goals. I found that yoga provided me with a more perceptive outlook on life. My new choices were based on a more profound self-awareness and a fresh sense of priorities. Yoga is an approach offering many options or roads to take. Your destination is a matter of choice. However, it's the journey there that counts.

The First Cut Is the Deepest

The first time I signed up for a yoga class—thirty-odd years ago—I walked into the room and felt like the odd man out. I know that for a large percentage of women, especially those over twenty-five, it takes a lot of guts to show up for an exercise class wearing a leotard. You feel like you need to work out first, before even starting the class. Likewise, as I took my place in the room, I felt extremely awkward. Faces turned to look at me, check me out . . . and, worst of all, recognize me. I asked myself what the hell I was doing here. But quickly decided, *I might as well see it through.*

The charismatic yoga master, Bikram Choudhury, conducted the class in a preheated room and expertly guided us through deep breathing, followed by a series of pretty strenuous aerobic standing postures. My heart was pounding, and I realized yoga could also provide a cardio workout! This was followed by floor postures to strengthen and lengthen the spine, a great antidote to "dowager's hump" and shrinking height. I started breathing hard, and my muscles trembled with the effort. Fortunately, each time I felt winded, the sequence would change, which served to balance out my system and revitalize me. By the time class ended, I lay there completely restored. I walked out of there feeling three feet off the ground, buoyant, and in a great mood! This was a switch, since I'd left home that morning in a blue funk. Already the benefits were evident. I was hoping it wasn't a fluke, because nothing outside of a stiff cup of European-blend coffee had ever given me such a boost before . . . and *this* was "on the natch," as in *natural high*.

Three decades later, I credit yoga with a more youthful appearance, even in my late sixties, along with a sense of serenity, vitality, and an enriching spiritual awareness. Oh—and I'm able to meditate now!

Clearing Emotional Blocks

Yoga was also instrumental in guiding me gently through what I call emotional "blocks," by which I mean pockets of trapped emotion that inhibit the functioning of your internal organs; feelings like fear, sadness, anger, resentment, frustration, and just about any intense emotion you can think of. These *blocks* can also come from childhood memories or unresolved problems that have wounded your psyche. Such experiences accumulate over time, sometimes years, and are stored in the living tissues of the body.

They interfere with circulation in various internal organs and form "scars" (my metaphor) inside your body and mind. These accumulated memories are sometimes the result of experiences that have been repeated over and over . . . as history tends to repeat itself.

How can we break the cycle? The answer is by systematically breaking up the blocks and sweeping them clean from the body and mind. I think we all stuff back emotions almost on a daily basis. Although we feel things strongly, we're unable to "act out" everything we feel, and for good reason. We'd all end up in the loony bin. You know the axiom, "Life is a *tragedy* for those who feel but a *comedy* for those who think."

My own personal experience may better illustrate what I'm talking about in regard to clearing emotional blocks. As a novice, only about three weeks into my practice, I was performing one of those impossible postures—the Standing Head to Knee pose. I was thinking, *I'll never do this one.* Despite my pessimism, I found myself executing the pose perfectly! Once I settled into position, I held the pose for close to a minute, controlling my breath and balance. I didn't know it then, but I was on the verge of a breakthrough. With an almost imperceptible shift, I felt something release . . . nothing big or jarring; something incredibly subtle, but deep . . . and suddenly my breathing became easier. I sensed a euphoric out-of-body lightness, as if I were not *doing* the pose . . . I was just *in* it . . . poised in a moment of effortless perfection. Involuntarily, without any warning, tears started to flow . . . a steady silent stream dropping very softly onto the floor. Nobody even noticed but me. A weight had been lifted from my heart, and with every fiber of my being, I could feel myself emerging, rather like a butterfly emerges from its chrysalis.

This moment of rebirth seemed much more valuable than the physical "buffing," that had been my original motive for taking up yoga. Not long after that, I realized that all the emotional blocks I'd felt as an actress when I was trying to access my emotions had been dissolved away. Words cannot describe the joy I felt to be relieved of this burden, which had probably been building up since childhood, made worse by the price of fame.

Attitude Is Everything

If you choose yoga, you will need a steady, consistent approach to achieve visible results in approximately thirty days. It's best in the learning stage to take a class or practice every day. Gulp! In this way the muscle memory and coordination required for the postures will become second nature. You will achieve very encouraging signs even after the first week or ten days if you practice regularly without a break. After this beginning period, you may decide to *yogacize* every other day. Most people are so impressed with how they feel and look that they choose to continue with their practice five or six days a week.

Like all new physical or mental pursuits, the beginning stage is the most challenging and difficult; and with age you must battle against those self-critical comparisons with how you performed in younger days. Those comparisons and our tendency to look back instead of forward will undermine your efforts. Please, do not inflict judgment on yourself and become negative. It's perfectly natural to be awkward and inept when you're learning something new.

I began my yoga practice when I was in my late thirties. Clearly, how I performed then was influenced by my youth. Now, in my sixties, my approach is out of necessity quite different, and it has helped me accept how I must adjust to the passing years by changing my strategy. My approach now is based more on a mental, spiritual level and I have had to learn to be patient (not my forte) and move more slowly toward my goals. Fortunately, slow and steady works just as well. Nonetheless, I've had to accept that postures I once took pride in performing perfectly are now ones that I struggle with. But struggle I must, and even though it takes longer, in the end I surprise myself. Faithful commitment and working at your own level, without regret, does it every time . . . from your thirties to your sixties and beyond. Bikram likes to say, "You're never too young, never too old, never too sick, and it's never too late to begin yoga."

I became even more convinced of that and of the anti-aging benefits of yoga when I witnessed my own mother take up this practice for the first time at age sixty-five! I watched with trepidation, since she suffered from an arthritic knee and could hardly walk. What guts! I was worried because I'd never known her to do anything very physical, except work hard around the house and garden. "I used to swim, darling, when I was a schoolgirl," she once offered. But there she was, coming to class every day without fail. I was so proud of her. She'd always stand in the back row and sometimes hold onto a ballet bar for support and balance. Mom didn't seem to mind that the much younger students could do all the postures better than she could. She was always smiling and, oh boy, she sure didn't give up . . . not once. I use her as inspiration when I attend yoga class these days.

After a month or so, her knee improved and she no longer walked with a limp; the swelling in her lower joints subsided and she didn't complain any longer about pain. Plus she looked about ten years younger! She was delighted to notice that the fine lines on her face were smoothed away. She had good color without makeup and her eyes were bright and clear. I get a lump in my throat just thinking about her. She was really something and lived to be ninety-two.

No matter your age, once you train your muscle memory and co-ordination, you will be very well served in the future; because, like riding a bicycle, you can always go back and revisit this method as time marches on. Your younger friends are going to notice the difference in you. So why not suggest it to them, or to your children?

A healthy mental attitude is everything! But then, you knew that, didn't you? You're probably never going to start a health and fitness regimen unless your mind and heart are in the right place. "Keep thy heart with all diligence for out of it springs the issues of life." (Proverbs 4:23)

I believe that the heart works through the prism of the imagination, which is most fertile in young children. We tend to get cynical as we mature and lose that hopeful innocence. But our inner child never dies. We all have one. Naughty or nice, he or she is there beneath the surface directing our actions . . . and thank God that child is wired to our inner voice. What we often lose is the ability to listen to, hear, and acknowledge that voice, without being reminded to do so. Allow your inner child to be hopeful again. Imagine how you want to be and allow that urge to become a strong desire. Follow it.

The Breath of Life

Life begins with the breath and so it is in yoga. A single breath is the beginning of life and the underlying thread on which every thought, action, and emotion is supported or suspended. It is said that when you can control your breathing, you can control your emotions, and when you can control your emotions, life will cease to be a battlefield. The

Latin blessing *In spiritus sancto* refers to the sacred breath, or spirit. The breath and the spirit are clearly related.

For me, part of the appeal of yoga is how it's attuned to the ebb and flow of the universe that surrounds us. I think of yoga as a dance of life and find comfort in the physical poise that comes with it. With practice, your heart and lungs and your physical movements operate in sync; like Lance Armstrong atop his bicycle or Michael Phelps gliding through the water. It's so exhilarating when you come to that moment when everything becomes effortless for the first time. It really seems like a miracle. So every yoga session should begin with *deep breathing*. Once you've mastered it, you can even do it at home upon awaking. Like a moveable feast, you can partake of it wherever you go. Deep breathing is portable. Think of your breath as a barometer of mood swings. Tap into it secretly, even in a crowd, and refresh yourself whenever needed. Slip away to a deserted hallway and breathe deeply to calm your nerves. In addition to breathing, there are a lot of stretches and postures you can use outside of the yoga classroom. They can become yours to own. So just breathe.

Spiritual Benefits

As a final note, let me add that Hatha yoga is not in itself a religion, though it is often associated with Eastern mysticism, Hinduism, and Buddhism. I was raised Christian, and I continue to practice my faith; I do not see yoga as being in conflict with my principles. I see it as a comprehensive approach to health and wellness. If anything, it was instrumental in opening the way for me to rediscover my Christian faith. By the time I left home at eighteen, my belief was already wavering. I vaguely accepted by rote that there was a God, I just wasn't sure about the nature of such a being. I then became influenced by the changing values of the '60s. Swept along by the youth culture of the day, I started to seriously doubt whether there really was a God after all. I didn't want to explore those doubts, but I found nothing in my life experience nor in the hedonistic philosophy of the '60s that could rebut the disturbing question that glared at me from the cover of *Time* magazine, "Is God Dead?" (1966) If this was true, what code of ethics should I then follow? I could only look to my moral upbringing, which kept me away from what I'd been taught was bad behavior.

More than a decade later, when I ventured into hatha yoga, my classes didn't include any spiritual training or religious dogma whatsoever. My approach to yoga began as strictly physical, with mental benefits. However, as yoga worked to condition my senses, there came a point when I was able to come to the *realization* that I was a creature in God's universe and that I was only one small part of it. I came to a place of contentment and serenity, as though a great weight had been lifted from my shoulders; and I felt liberated in the knowledge that God does exist. I knew with certainty that I had experienced His presence, and I received this newly found surety with a flood of relief. I knew intuitively that I could "Let go and let God," as long as I was connected to my conscience, intuition, and a higher sense of right.

Like many of you, I've had difficulties with keeping true to that belief. But that is another subject. At this point, suffice it to say that the personal "temple" of my spirit was ready to be inhabited by something other than my own desires, fears, anger, and ego. How about you?

Yes, a woman reaching forty and moving past it into her fifties and sixties still faces a path full of obstacles. There are many social pressures that undermine her ability to thrive in later years and new challenges to prepare for and surmount. I encourage you to face any roadblocks head-on, with the knowledge that they may ultimately lead to the most fulfilling stage of your life.

SEVEN

Food and Your Body Image

I CONSIDER EATING FOR FUN AND FLAVOR one of the joys of living, but if I ate everything that my appetite dictates, I'd blow up like the Goodyear Blimp. Around my fifty-fifth year, I started to notice that my metabolism burned calories at a different rate and that my digestive system worked less efficiently. I also discovered that I wasn't really assimilating all the important, life-sustaining nutrients from my food, so I was wilting on the vine. In a sense, I was starving for certain crucial elements. It was a wake-up call for a new philosophy of eating. In other words, it was time to rethink my diet.

The subject of food and dieting immediately brings to mind *body image*. As a woman, I've spent a lifetime tied to such concerns, along with the fear and anxiety they bring. It's a highly emotional battlefield for most women, and I'm no exception. Sometimes, when I *need* to be body conscious for professional reasons, it's like dragging around a ball and chain. The obligation weighs heavily on me, and I am not truly free to follow my impulses. Though food is not on my mind constantly, I take pains not to let more than ten pounds come between me and my ideal weight. It's a necessary burden, if I want to look good in my favorite clothes.

Back in the day, *I* had *the* body that intimidated most women, and some of you probably even hated me for it. And now, here I am, squirming at the sight of those gorgeous but impossibly thin models. Body issues were already oppressive enough in my twenties. At sixty-nine, the pressure is off the hook! I'm also sensitive to the fact that the fashion industry deliberately designs clothes that discriminate against those who don't fit into that particular mold. But remind myself *constantly* that it's a woman's prerogative whether to bow in submission to these trends *or not.*

Will I back off and retreat? No, I won't. I don't intend to let fashion dictate what I should look like, but I don't want to drop out of the "marathon," so to speak, before crossing the finish line. I suspect that most women wrestle with that problem on a daily basis. It seems none of us is immune.

Actually, I faced a lot of rejection when I first came to Hollywood. I got turned down at every modeling agency in town. They said I was the wrong shape . . . so much for all those beauty contests. I didn't fit the prototype that was "in" that year. I hung around like the runt of the litter until I landed a hand commercial. My hands and feet were pretty, so I was able to model shoes as well. But they weren't interested in the rest of me.

I finally found a job in the garment district as a fitting model, but was never allowed to walk the runway. I was confined to a back room where they pinned muslin patterns on me. Every day I heard complaints about my physical proportions. Shoulders too broad, hips not right, waist too thin, bosom too full; and with each gripe came an irritated tug on the muslin that was pinned around my body, jerking me this way and that. After six months of being pushed, pulled, and pinched, I was reduced to a pretty low opinion of myself. But I stuck it out. I needed the money to buy a car and pay for a babysitter.

In the ensuing years, I managed to break through as an actress and landed a ten-year movie contract at 20th Century Fox, the home of Marilyn Monroe and Betty Grable, no less. There I fit right in. This time, I had people actually believing, or fooled into thinking, that I was a real looker! Damn, don'tcha love it? But if I've learned anything during the four decades I've spent trading on my body image, it's this: Don't take any of it too seriously . . . not the praise nor the rejection. It's all just a game!

Curb Your Eating Habits

I reject ephedrine, smoking, bulimia, and other such desperate measures to lose weight. I've always been a health addict. It's the only thing I know that works for me. And though it takes some willpower and discipline, it's very liberating to find yourself in control. It's extremely hard to break bad eating habits once they've become ingrained, but it is definitely possible. The desire for health and longevity, weight loss, vitality and an attractive physical appearance demands that, like it or not, we need to address the problem and get motivated.

As a kid I loved pancakes and waffles sprinkled with powdered sugar and warm syrup. There were always cookies, pies, and pastries in our house and freshly baked cinnamon rolls for breakfast. *Yummmmm . . . slurp.*

I wasn't a big fan of vegetables. But even in my twenties, when I began making movies and often appeared in swimsuits, miniskirts, and other figure-conscious clothes, I had to ditch the morning doughnuts. It was a *huge* sacrifice, especially when I was away from home and living alone in a hotel room I *needed* that doughnut! That sweet consoling taste became the symbol of everything I was forced to sacrifice to be in the movies. But of course I *had* to resist my sweet tooth; I couldn't afford to crack. Weighing everything in the balance—including the doughnuts— I came to the conclusion that the trade-off was worth it. It boiled down to the fact that I'd rather savor the sweet satisfaction I get from my career and lifestyle than indulging in fattening foods. So I streamlined my eating habits to support the life I'd chosen, and I vowed to keep my diet in check. It was my choice.

Have you ever noticed that when you're mentally engaged in some activity, you forget to eat? Does that tell you something? Overeating has become more of a compensation for emotional needs than a means of ingesting nutritional fuel.

Knowing how to eat properly will bring a positive change to your life. You'll enter a whole new world where you're not a slave to your cravings. You can and will start taking charge of your life.

For most of my life I ate what everyone else was eating and thought that if I didn't feel good there must be something wrong with *me*. Eventually I realized that I was different, and after consulting a recommended nutritionist, I learned to eat what was right for me. Like many teenagers, I ate cheeseburgers, fries, and chocolate shakes on the weekends. But after high school, when I became pregnant with my first child, I quickly cleaned up my act and became very careful about diet. Besides expecting a baby at such a young age, I was also doing that morning television show in San Diego called *Sun Up!* As the weather girl I had to rise and shine before dawn each morning. I used to wake up at 4 AM . . . throw up . . . try to eat something, ugh . . . dress . . . do my makeup . . . throw up . . . drive to the studio . . . have a doughnut (that's all they had) . . . throw up . . . get the weather report off the AP and UP wire services . . . try soda crackers . . . write my notes . . . throw up and, finally, manage to be bright-eyed for the cameras, after which I would once again . . . throw up! It was pretty daunting, and I was buckling under the strain. But it never occurred to me that this taxing schedule, the wear and tear on my nerves, plus my pregnancy, would affect my digestion. Ordinarily, I might have slid by on sheer adrenaline, but this time it was too tough on me.

In addition to having morning sickness, I was not yet aware that I was allergic to wheat and had an over-acidic stomach that reacted badly to raw food. I would have been better off if I'd been eating baby food *myself* while awaiting my first child. At any rate, I had a beautiful baby boy, Damon, seven pounds, seven ounces. Despite my initial weight loss from morning sickness, my son was very healthy and energetic. He was so robust that I had to attach shock absorbers to the legs of his crib! I had only managed to gain fourteen pounds during my pregnancy. But I still wasn't aware of the underlying problems inherent in my digestive system that contributed to my queasy stomach. By the time I had my second baby, two years later, my adorable daughter Tahnee, I think I held the world record for staring at the bottom of a toilet bowl. But happily, for nearly thirty years now, I've eaten a nutritionist-designed diet that balances out my stomach acids, and I'm absolutely fine.

Customize Your Diet

I learned everything I know about food from Eileen Poole, a wonderful nutritionist who has become a trusted friend. It has now been twenty-nine years since she reshaped my life through a customized diet. Until then it was trial and error. I'd never gone to a doctor to lose weight, but because of all those swimsuits, I was always interested in shedding a few pounds. Have you been there? However, good looks are not the only criterion of a good diet.

I wasn't feeling well when I came to Eileen. I'd been suffering with daily abdominal cramps and painful bloating after meals, and I was losing energy. Eileen discovered quickly that certain food combinations, thought of as "healthy" for most people, were *not indicated* for me. I apparently didn't fit into the norm again. I mean, who does?

Eileen redesigned my entire "diet"—she doesn't like that word, because she says it sounds so temporary and that eating should be *a way of life*. I agree! She said I should avoid starches like potatoes and bread and concentrate on steamed green veggies. I was to choose asparagus over carrots, have broccoli instead of corn. *Et voilà!* Within two weeks of changing my eating habits, I was on my way to feeling like a new woman! She proved to me that what is good for one person is not necessarily good for another. Your customized diet, besides serving your nutritional needs, should eliminate those harmful foods that trigger allergies and threaten the efficiency of your digestive system. If you give it a chance to work, a proper diet can relieve almost any unhealthy symptoms and give you a tremendous feeling of well-being. I'm such a believer that I sent both my children to Eileen years ago, so that they, too, could gain the benefits of eating correctly, within their own individual needs.

Just a reminder: A diet has physical *and* mental components. There is a mind-body connection when it comes to nutrition too. A balanced diet will help you on both fronts.

My Food Bag

I find that the best way to deal with meals is to *plan ahead*, especially if you're starting a new diet. Planning ahead is also helpful if you're getting back on the wagon after a cheating binge. The idea is to have regular breaks where you eat the right foods in the right portions and combinations. Most of my meals are three to four hours apart, with mini snacks in between and no meals after six o'clock. This may entail preparing food in advance, but it's pretty easy, and you'll get used to it. Think of it as the lunch bag you used to carry to school. It's easier in New York or in closely knit urban centers to just stop by a small neighborhood deli, but that's a bit dangerous for me! All that gorgeous food looks pretty inviting! I'm not immune to display cases full of sumptuous temptations. So, to help me with my vows of abstinence, I rely on my food bag to steer me away from cheating.

I pack water, an apple, rice cakes, and a light meal that will fit into a small plastic container, such as sliced chicken with, say, steamed asparagus. My bag has pockets for plastic forks, straws, condiments, napkins, etc. I just put it behind the seat in my car and I'm off to the hairdresser, shopping, or wherever I need to go throughout the day. Eating out is a special occasion . . . but being forced to stop in the middle of my errands to buy junk food is a sure way to ruin my resolve. There are too many goodies in the food court, and I don't even want to *see* a menu! I'm not made of steel!

Fresh Start

Start your new diet in a time period like a free weekend, when you can concentrate on changing your routine. There's no question that there will be an adjustment period, when you alter your eating habits and adopt a schedule that you're not accustomed to. Get ready for it. Regular eating times and prescribed low-cal snacks are super important. If you don't stay the course, you will likely end up eating late at night, when we're all prone to binge. The following morning, you'll wake up with a food hangover and a sluggish start to the day. Plus, as you well know, eating late at night just before you retire is the worst time, because you go to bed soon after and therefore don't burn as many calories! That doesn't work in my profession. Once late-night eating takes hold, it's a vicious circle, prompting your whole sleep cycle to fall later and later until, there you are, munching after midnight while staring mindlessly at late-night television! Believe me, I've been there, surrounded by potato chip remnants and a dose of Alka-Seltzer to treat the damage. Not a pretty sight.

I hate to sound like a taskmaster, but the true secret behind enviable beauty is hard work and discipline. If you're willing, it all pays off. You can become your own makeover project. There are two things that I recommend to support you in your efforts. First, invest in a gym membership or find a workout buddy who's an early riser to share your morning walk or workout, so there's no room for excuses. If you can afford it, get a reliable cardio machine and hit it every day, even when it's dark outside or the weather is bad. Second, hook up with a qualified nutritionist, who can design a customized eating program, just for you. Most "diets" end up being temporary solutions—they're often unsustainable. It is well worth the expense (approximately $200) to get yourself a personalized diet designed by a qualified nutritionist. What you gain is a plan that will control your weight, boost your energy, and give you the proper nutrition you deserve. If the spirit is willing and you can bend the flesh to your will, you absolutely *can* maintain your health and look great as you get older.

Food Is Your Best Medicine

I've been around since the Dinosaur Age, so I've had more than enough time to note that the Western medical profession, with few exceptions, has been slow to understand the correlation between food and disease (both physical and mental). There's nothing new about this connection. On the contrary, it's fundamental. It's true that for several decades there have been numerous medical studies covering the connection between nutrition and disease, but their important findings didn't make a sizable enough impact on popular culture; and in my opinion, they failed to emphasize the curative powers of a prescribed diet to treat specific diseases. The obvious benefits of certain pharmaceutical remedies and surgical techniques should not obscure what we know to be organically sound; namely, that *good food is the best preventive medicine.* If you abuse your body through improper diet (what is inappropriate for you), it will pave the way for diseases of every variety, from cancer to heart disease to emphysema. An excellent book on this subject is *Food Is Your Best Medicine*, by the nutrition pioneer Henry G. Bieler, M.D.

Years ago, I received a bulletin from the American Institute for Cancer Research, issuing the following statement: "Breast cancer may be prevented and perhaps even controlled through proper diet. Experts now estimate that 60 percent of the cancer in women *may* be caused by consistently eating the wrong diet." Pretty mind-blowing! It stands to reason that, if improper diet can create a toxic climate in the body that invites disease, the reverse is also true: That disease can be "cured," or at least arrested by a proper diet. The use of drugs and surgery may be necessary, but preferably as a last resort. Clearly, no surgeon is eager to perform unnecessary and risky procedures, nor is any reputable physician keen on prescribing drugs, with their accompanying side effects, before all other avenues have been explored. But it is also true that not enough doctors are well versed in the virtues of nutritional cures. My hope is that the new trend toward body awareness will encourage a more organic approach toward disease and well-being. Currently, such remedies are still reduced to the category of "alternative medicine."

The Battle of the Bulge

Countless women have asked about my personal diet, but when I tell them, they protest that they could never go through such "torture." In a nutshell, besides abstaining from salt, sugar, and caffeine, I stick to a lo-carb, hi-protein approach. Basically, a meal consists of 4 ounces of protein and includes as many steamed green lo-carb veggies I want. I also allow myself three fruits per day or I can substitute a 4-ounce glass of juice. For breakfast I have egg whites or a non-wheat grain and try to avoid dairy products and preservatives. Most people would balk. It reminds me of the first time I heard that the likes of Bette Davis, Ginger Rogers, and Marilyn Monroe had all submitted to a crushing schedule of sixteen hours a day. I was stunned! The same kind of commitment is also required when starting a diet, especially one with transformative potential.

When my goal is to lose weight, I usually need to be motivated by some outside influence that sparks me to want to get in shape. Once I begin the process, it becomes enjoyable to monitor my progress as a sleeker body emerges from its fleshy cocoon of sloth and gluttony. One can almost become addicted to the whole process. Somewhere deep within our feminine nature there lives a female warrior, and when necessary, she can be summoned to action. Hop to it, girls.

My Diet Guidelines

I can't recommend my diet regimen to everyone. It was, after all, prescribed particularly for me; but you might glean something from the eating principles I follow, which are key to many effective weight control programs. In any case, no diet worth its (lack of) salt is something to jump into lightly. There are many factors, like blood type, body type, and lifestyle, which affect digestion and the specific nutrients you need.

In order to effectively reeducate your taste buds, cleanse your entire digestive system, and pave the way for the reintroduction of *certain* foods back into your diet, please take note of the method of eating described below. I highly recommend these principles to any woman over forty, which is when I adopted this way of eating. If you've already hit fifty or even sixty and fallen into bad habits, you're not alone. It just takes a little time and resolve to adjust. In either case, keep sight of your goal, knowing that healthy eating habits can help you drop unwanted pounds, unlock vital energy, waken your senses, and increase your mental clarity. Oh, and you'll look great, too!

Food combining is an essential part of my personalized diet. Any good cook knows that the choice of ingredients, how you combine them and in what proportions make all the difference. The same thing applies to your daily diet. The term *food combining* deals with what *combinations* of foods work best to aid digestion and weight loss. It's easy once you get the hang of it. There are only two main rules to follow:

Rule 1: Do not mix protein and carbohydrates at the same meal.

For example, if you decide on pasta for your main course, choose a *nonprotein* marinara sauce —*without meat*; and eliminate grated cheese (it's a protein). You may also have *low-starch* vegetables like asparagus, spinach, broccoli, green beans, zucchini, summer squash and yellow squash, artichokes, and snow peas (to name a few of my favorites); but *skip the meat, poultry, or fish in a meal of carbohydrates.* Usually, the portion of pasta for small- to medium-size women is ¾ cup uncooked. You can make up for that with all the low-starch green vegetables you want.

The other option is to decide on a protein (fish, poultry, or lean meat) for the main course. The portion is a quarter pound. In this case, skip the pasta or potatoes and bring on a generous portion of *low-starch* vegetables again, or a green salad. Simple, isn't it?

If you choose to have a salad with your meat, *make it a green salad.* Avoid the cheese, avocados (high in fat), olives (ditto), tomatoes (classified as a fruit because they have a higher sugar content than most veggies). Don't add extra protein beyond the quarter pound allowed. Or you can make a meal of a large green salad alone, without any protein. Olive oil and lemon or vinegar is best for dressing.

Rule 2: Do not mix fruit (high in sugar content) with vegetables or with protein at the same meal.

The only exception to this rule is apples, which seem to combine with most foods. It's best to eat your fruit separately. Wait at least half an hour after a meal, or eat fruit as a snack between meals. It is all right to eat a small single portion (1 cup) of baked fruit with some starches, such as with your morning cereal. In fact, it's better than using sugar.

Generally speaking, you can't go wrong by following these food combining principles. Special exceptions to the rule are best prescribed by a doctor or a qualified nutritionist.

Cheating

People always ask if I ever break down and cheat. Yes, of course. Though I hate to admit it, I've been known to devour an entire homemade apple pie at a single sitting. I just can't stand the thought of that pie sitting there uneaten all night long. It haunts my dreams! But *usually* I'm very disciplined. For example, when I first started out, I managed to stay on my prescribed diet for three years solid before pigging out. It must be some kind of a record, but truthfully, it really wasn't much of a sacrifice. For most people, this new way of eating is easy to learn. It's something you never forget, and if you fall off the wagon you can always get right back on track.

Once I had reeducated my taste buds, I started to discover the natural flavor of food for the very first time. *Deeelicious!* The original taste of food is often overwhelmed by salts, spices, and other seasonings, such as MSG, which are easy to become addicted to. Once you sample the real thing, additives are like gilding the lily. I just ate fresh, lightly steamed snow peas and broccoli for lunch. *Sooo good*.

I would never encourage you to be casual about following your personalized eating plan. But if you should sneak in a "side" of fries, or maybe a piece of chocolate cake, don't beat yourself up over it. Usually, after the first two weeks of any diet, the urge to cheat is gone. So make a deal with yourself that you absolutely *will not cheat* for at least two weeks. No excuses. Getting off to a good start is crucial. After a successful launch, you'll be in orbit.

Damage Control

Every once in a while a girl may need a little reliable damage control. We all slip up by indulging in sugars and starches, and when we do, the after-effects can play havoc with our kidneys, spleen, pancreas, and liver. The best remedy I can recommend to rebalance the alkaline in your system and recover from a sugar hangover is Bieler's Broth, formulated by Dr. Henry Bieler. This puree-of-vegetable soup is my all-purpose best friend when I'm feeling low. I also drink it the morning after a culinary indiscretion. Unfortunately, there is no effective fix for regular bouts of cheating, but this soothing soup works as a temporary reprise. It's also the solution I use to avoid getting discouraged and falling still further into bingeing. In addition, Bieler's Broth can be used in place of meals when fasting. It's nourishing and calming because it's loaded with more vitamins and minerals than other fasting or cleansing drinks. I drink it almost daily in place of a veggie, and it's particularly good when you're feeling stressed or have indigestion. I keep a supply on hand in the fridge, because it's beneficial in endless ways.

Anytime you feel low, sluggish, or run-down and on the verge of catching something like a cold or the flu, this is an excellent deterrent. I haven't had a dose of antibiotics in years! Although Bieler's Broth is not a gourmet treat, I've come to enjoy the subtle flavor of this saltless, creamless, spiceless soup. When you experience how good you feel, it begins to taste pretty darn good. It's also good for a hangover.

Bieler's Broth recipe

Place 1 quart water in a deep saucepan and bring to a boil. Now add the following ingredients: 1 pound string beans (strings removed), 3 medium-size zucchini (sliced), 1 medium-size bunch of parsley (without stems), 2 stalks of celery, with the strings removed. (It's easy to strip the outside of the celery stalk by hand, with a potato peeler, or with a paring knife, and it's worth the extra 30 seconds of preparation to avoid celery strings in your soup.) You'll find that celery has a remarkable cleansing effect on the colon.

Let these veggies cook until medium tender (approximately five minutes). Be careful not to overcook, or you will lose most of the nutrients. When the vegetables are ready, remove them from the water with a slotted spoon and place in a blender. Be sure to *save the water, because it has absorbed a lot of the nutrients from the vegetables*. Use an appropriate amount of cooked veggies, leaving enough room to add that vitamin-rich water. Blend to the consistency of pea soup. Test for your desired thickness before passing the point of no return. Some people like more crunch than others. Add more water if it's too thick. Remember, once you start the blending phase, you cannot remove the water. If your blended broth is a rich hunter green, that's a good sign. If the broth looks pale green or army green, chances are you've overcooked your ingredients. Good luck and good health!

Vitamin Supplements

We would be better able to get the *full nutritional value* from the food we eat if it were not subjected to modern techniques that compromise the quality of our produce and livestock. Unfortunately, much of the food available to us is processed. There are, however, a growing number of health food markets nationwide where organically grown, hormone-free foods are available. Nonetheless, as we age, *nutritional supplements become essential.* Fortunately, there are many clinically tested and easily assimilated supplements that can augment what we need as we grow older. My personal choices are listed below:

✓ Triple Joint Formula—glucosamine, chondroitin, and MSM, for joint health.

✓ Calcium—1200 milligrams per day, divided equally over three meals, to help prevent osteoporosis.

✓ Magnesium—Take in pure ionic form to maximize absorption. Magnesium is assimilated in the body only after it is ionized by hydrochloric acid (HCL). As we age, we produce progressively lower levels of this acid.

✓ Vitamin C—with D, rose hips, bioflavonoids, and rutin. I take 3000 milligrams per day divided between meals for support of blood vessels, adrenal glands, and the immune system.

✓ Vitamin B-12 complex—Take regularly as part of a multivitamin regimen or, when under performance stress and long hours, one submuscular injection daily (consult your physician before using injectable supplements); also available in extract form.

✓ Vitamin E with selenium—400 milligrams per day.

✓ Armour Thyroid—This is a natural product for hormone replacement therapy, not a synthetic compound. It provides both of the key thyroid hormones.

✓ DHEA—For adrenal support, take 5 milligrams once per day before late afternoon.

✓ Licorice root—solid extract at a 5:1 ratio, ¼ teaspoon, three times a day, for low adrenals; must be ordered from a compounding pharmacy.

✓ Probiotics—Buy a triple superstrain formula—with acidophilus, bifidus, and bulgaricus; and take one capsule each morning with meals. Maintains low-pH levels and supplies beneficial bacteria to support the immune system.

✓ Black cohosh—a tincture that comes in a small bottle with a dropper; good for hot flashes.

✓ Green Tea Extract—another tincture with dropper; supports healthy pancreas, fat levels, and cholesterol that are already within the normal range. Promotes high antioxidant activity as well as healthy connective tissue and joint flexibility.

✓ Flaxseed meal—helps control cholesterol levels and is an excellent source of fiber. I sprinkle it on my cereal or mix it in a protein drink at least once a day.

✓ Psyllium husk capsules—for added fiber.

✓ Digestive enzymes

✓ Shen Min—a Chinese herbal tablet for hair and nails.

To ensure that these key nutrients are assimilated effectively, vitamins should be taken with meals and at the recommended daily dosage. Be aware that vitamins A, D, E, and K have been shown to cause negative side effects if taken in excess. In fact, A, D, and E are all oil-soluble and can't pass out of the body as easily as the water-soluble vitamins B and C. So consult your doctor for recommendations.

Most health-conscious women today already take supplements and watch their diets, but every small detail I've included to combat aging has proved important and valuable to my quality of life. Now is not the time to slack off or resign ourselves to the notion that we cannot fight the inevitable. I can only tell you that each time I neglect to exercise, eat right, and take my supplements, I feel a marked difference, and it's more pronounced than when I was younger. This may seem like too much to remember, but even the smallest thing plays an important part. To quote Mies van der Rohe, "God is in the details."

Part III

HOW
YOU
LOOK

EIGHT

The Skin You're In

SKIN IS THE SEXY, HIGHLY SENSITIVE WRAP-per that covers your body's entire surface. It makes up the largest organ of the human body. It also very accurately reflects the state of your health inside and out. Because of that, I've always had a great deal of respect for the care and feeding of my skin. I inherited my fine-pored complexion from my mother and took my cue from her about how I should treat it. I paid close attention to how she first moisturized her face and then applied her makeup. She put the same moisturizer on again each night. This set the pattern that I would follow my whole life. It became my personal ritual.

My mother used an affordable moisturizer from the drugstore, Oil of Olay, and I followed suit, never changing to any other formula from age fifteen to sixty-nine. This proved to me that you don't have to buy expensive creams and lotions for your skin to look radiant. Although I've tried other products, nothing seems to suit my cellular makeup quite as well as my original tried-and-true moisturizer. I don't stick with it just because my mother used it, because believe me, I didn't follow her example when it came to a zillion other things; but when I slather on a coat of Olay, without fail, my skin sits up and takes notice. It seems to just drink it in, as though savoring a favorite treat.

Though I subscribe to the benefits of spa treatments and facials, I am often pressed for time and do not have the luxury of indulging in these pleasures as often as I might like. While on location for many years, I learned how to be self-sufficient when it comes to skin care. Out of necessity, I have become well acquainted with over-the-counter do-it-yourself facials, which I give myself every other week, in the privacy of my own home. It doesn't take long. The home treatment I use is my old standby, Olay Regenerist, a two-step system using derma-crystals, followed by activator serum.

What can I tell you? I'm pretty self-reliant and down-to-earth when you get to know me. I've always taken care of my skin using a very straightforward method and a formula that goes back decades. It's nothing costly or exotic, but it works like gangbusters. The secret is, I moisturize every day, both morning and evening. Just like consistent exercise, it pays off.

A Nightly Ritual

Most would agree that the tone and texture of your skin is the single most important factor in a youthful appearance. This is especially true for your face, neck, and décolletage. No matter what your age—the younger you start, the better—the need to care for your skin daily is essential.

Did you know that your skin breathes? It also eats and is dying to be fed every day. Your hungry skin soaks up anything that comes into contact with its surface, whether it be water, sunlight, air, moisturizer, or medication, either ingested or in the form of a transdermal patch. Not only is it affected by what you eat, it's affected by your hormones. Your skin needs to be nourished, and it requires a diet, too. It also responds well to the increased blood circulation that comes with exercise. All these things affect the skin dramatically.

Like I said, I'm a fanatic about applying moisturizers. It comes as second nature to me because I've been doing it for so many years. First,

I remove my makeup with old-fashioned hypoallergenic cleansing milk, which hardly anyone makes anymore. Thanks to Clarins, I can still find it. I apply the cleanser all over my face and neck. Then I wet a washcloth and wring it out, so that it's damp but not dripping. With this damp cloth, I remove the cream from my face and neck gently without dragging the cloth across the skin. Then I rinse off any excess cleanser with tap water, using my hands and fingers only. I pat my skin dry, and while it's still damp, I apply moisturizer. Like clockwork I repeat this same ritual every night before I retire. A few years ago I developed my own skin-care formula, which was scheduled to launch nationally in the summer of 2002. However, the entire enterprise was aborted because of the 9/11 attacks. In the climate of fear that followed, it was next to impossible to market new products. The anthrax scare also killed mail-order deliveries. Maybe one day, I'll retrieve those formulas and start again.

Exposure to the sun can have a profound and lasting effect on the condition of your skin. I always wear a hat and sunblock to avoid exposing my face and décolletage directly to the sun. Even reflected rays can be damaging. However, I do believe that short periods of sun exposure can be both healthy and satisfying and can make you look attractive, if taken at the right hours when the sun is not high in the sky. On spring vacation, I've noticed that the sun is usually mild between 9 AM and 10 AM. Or late in the day, from 4 PM to 5 PM. The body can usually stand more exposure than the face, and on the beach I enjoy the feeling of the sea air and the relaxing sensation of soaking up all that warm, "preheated" vitamin D. Even so, if you do the same, be careful not to burn your arms, upper back, and shoulders. And be aware that summer sun is usually more brutal.

As I've already mentioned, to help combat signs of aging and sun damage, I also make use of biweekly gentle over-the-counter home facials, which I know will not burn or damage my complexion. I have very fine, sensitive skin, so I am extremely selective about the products and spa treatments I indulge in. I end up doing 90 percent of my skin-care maintenance at home. I do miss that lovely pampered feeling I get with a salon facial, but in the final analysis, for my needs, a good home treatment works quite well.

Caring for your skin at home is a practical solution for those of you who, like me, are pressed for time. It's also a lot less expensive. Since I'm now in my late sixties, understandably there have been those times when I've become discouraged by growing older and can identify with that sinking feeling that it's too late and I might as well pack it in. But if that's what you're feeling right now because you've neglected yourself for a while, let me assure you that it's never too late to start again. The body is remarkably resilient and always ready to reward a consistent effort. You can revive your aging skin with regular care. You just have to take the first step toward that goal and stick with it.

Anti-Wrinkle Patches

There are some old-fashioned methods that have been passed over in the past couple of decades in the stampede to the surgeon's office. One particular set of tricks I've used to great effect over the years dates back to the silent era of film. I hesitate to tell you about it, knowing there are those who are likely to dismiss anything not considered "cutting edge." But before you discount this trick, let me explain how this method came to my attention back in the '60s, when I was still in my twenties.

My second husband, Patrick Curtis, had a paternal aunt who was a real character. I've come to think of her as a petite version of Auntie Mame, because she appeared one afternoon dressed to the nines in a brightly colored sheath, with a handbag and hat to match. She was a flamboyant costume designer who worked for the studios. But what struck me as rather bizarre was that she was wearing these small, flesh-colored triangles on her face! She had one placed between her eyebrows, one near the outside corner of each eye, and two more like parentheses on either side of her mouth.

I actually managed to carry on a conversation with Auntie without mentioning the patches. Later on, I found out that they were called

THE SKIN YOU'RE IN

Frownies and had been around since the late nineteenth century. Then the time came in my early forties when I realized that, though I still looked good, it couldn't last forever. Ever the one to engage in preventive measures, I found the very same Frownies at a beauty supply store in New York and started using them that night. I've even used them on long flights beneath a sleep mask, or when I'm driving down the coast to visit my sister. But there are limits. Unlike Auntie, I don't like to wear them when other people are around and definitely not when Mr. Wonderful is close by.

You've likely never heard much about them because, like Auntie M in my story, they are ancient. And yet, I'm only one of many well-known actresses, models, and professional beauties who use this method, because it works! They really do help reduce wrinkling. Ranella Hirsch, M.D., a dermatologist, was quoted in Oprah Winfrey's magazine *O* as saying, "There are a few noninvasive steps you can take to reduce lines. I know a woman who swears by Frownies, little pieces of tape you can put on your frown areas at night when you go to sleep, to keep you from cultivating lines." Dr. Hirsch also recommends getting your eyes checked; you may not realize how often you're squinting, causing wrinkles to develop.

I have to confess that I was pretty darn skeptical when I first tried using Frownies. I couldn't forget the image of my eccentric Auntie Mame. But the proof was in the pudding. At almost seventy, I can't say that I am wrinkle free, but my skin looks amazingly good for my age. I'm not too proud to stick these little suckers on my face every night. But I stop short of getting all dolled up and walking out the door with them on!

Frownies work on a principle similar to Botox. Both methods prevent the facial muscle from contracting and leaving behind an imprint — a wrinkle. In the Botox method, a small amount of paralyzing poison is injected strategically into the skin, making the muscles "let go" and lines disappear. Frownies, on the other hand, act like a kind of splint to keep the muscle from contracting. The difference is that facial patches have a gradual, cumulative effect with continual use. The injection elicits an almost immediate reaction, but has to be repeated after several months. The other big difference is that Botox costs hundreds of dollars per treatment. Frownies cost $19 a box. Depending of course on how many patches are used per day, each box contains about a month's supply.

Back in the '70s, I met the awesome Gloria Swanson on a flight from Budapest to London. She was about seventy-five years old at the time and had not a line on her face. She was seated in the row directly opposite mine, so I had a clear view. After the safety belt sign flickered off, I noticed that she began to stick Frownie patches between her brows and next to her eyes. Then she put on a sleep mask and fell asleep.

When Gloria disembarked from the plane, the patches were gone and she skipped down the stairs with the energy of a twenty-five-year-old, looking absolutely great. (I found out later that she was a yogi, too!) We tend to think that we know so much more now than any previous generation, and yet, here is a simple and effective product with a long history!

Eye-Patch Therapy

Another area where you can ward off wrinkles at home during your regular skin-care regimen is the sensitive skin under the eyes. There are several eye-patch solutions that I've found to be very effective. They work with a transdermal delivery system that deposits a lipopeptide complex by means of crescent-shaped patches placed under each eye. Each patch contains a light gel formula that has been clinically proven to reduce fine lines and wrinkles under the eyes, resulting in a smooth, younger-looking appearance. Other transdermal patches offer formulas specifically for bags, dark circles, and puffiness under the eyes. Usually the patches come in a protective sealed packet. They have liners that easily peel off and help you place them under the eye. Leave these soothing patches on for twenty to forty minutes. Then remove gently and discard. I use mine once a week, and I always see an instant improvement.

I use this kind of therapy in the morning before a big event, or the night before. I wear them to bed if I have an early makeup call for work. Unlike the Frownies, they are soft and pliable. There are several different brands available that treat the under-eye area. You can find them on the Internet or in most drugstores.

Advanced Facial Treatments

Chemical peels   A chemical peel is a treatment in which alpha hydroxy acid (AHA) solution is used to remove the damaged outer layers of the skin. Typically administered as a facial, a chemical peel enhances and smooths the texture of the skin. It is an effective treatment for facial blemishes, wrinkles, and uneven skin pigmentation, without the use of an abrasive device. However, to make sure it's done safely, you may need more than one treatment. The technician should begin with a mild solution to determine the percentage of acid necessary to improve your skin without burning it. The downtime is minimal, so you should be able to return to work afterward. Facialists who are not medical personnel are only permitted to administer the less potent solutions, which are still quite effective.

My friend has done it on her lunch break! She repeats the treatment once every two weeks. The area will become red, and sunblock should be worn. Even with the sunblock, you should avoid direct exposure to the sun after the peel. Don't plan on going sailing, and use some common sense. Wear a hat and be extremely careful. How you treat the area will definitely affect the result. Those of you with olive skin, like me, may want to do a skin test on an area exposed to the sun, perhaps near your wrist, to ensure there will be no discoloration.

Much deeper peels are available, using stronger solutions such as trichloroacetic acid (TCA), most commonly used for medium-deep peeling, and phenol, which is the strongest of the chemical solutions and produces the deepest chemical peel. For these two stronger peels, you must consult a surgeon. To me, the mere thought of deep-burning the skin is a complete turnoff. It's definitely not on my to-do list.

Microdermabrasion   Even with my sensitive skin, I decided to try this treatment at a facial spa in Beverly Hills. They applied a solution to my face, and then they ran a special hand-held instrument in a circular motion over my skin. The process eliminates all the dead cells and also stimulates the production of new cells. Typically, there is no downtime, except that I was advised to stay out of the sun for twenty-four to forty-eight hours, which I did, and I used a sunblock under my makeup.

Scaredy cat that I am, they honored my request to go easy, because my skin is hypersensitive. The process was painless, and it gently exfoliated away the dead cells that had previously made my skin appear dull. Afterward, I was delighted that my skin really did look revitalized and rosy. They usually recommend a series of treatments for a cumulative effect over time. Depending on your skin requirements, you might want to try this particular treatment; it worked well for me.

Microdermabrasion used to be done with abrasive crystals. However, in the past decade, it has become more common to use a wand with a roughened surface. This is the method that was used successfully on my face. The procedure requires no medical monitoring and is commonly done by a trained esthetician in conjunction with other facial treatments.

Crystal and diamond microdermabrasion   Crystal microdermabrasion relies on tiny crystals that are sprayed onto the skin surface to perform the exfoliating process. Although the crystal microdermabrasion system is still widely used, the introduction of alternatives has led to a trend away from this treatment system. Diamond microdermabrasion—now the preferred method—operates in the same manner, but uses a diamond tipped tool rather than crystals.

Treatments at two-week intervals are recommended, and are often enough to maintain a radiant complexion. However, for more sturdy skin types with larger pores, more treatments might be necessary. I would say that it's best to try a couple of treatments first, before signing on for more than you actually need.

Laser resurfacing This is not a spa treatment. The procedure requires sedation and must be performed by a reputable surgeon. It eliminates the damaged surface layer of skin so your body will replace it with fresh skin cells. A wandlike laser makes the undesired skin cells and wrinkles literally disappear. One of the laser's most significant advantages over traditional techniques for skin resurfacing is that treatment is relatively bloodless. The procedure also offers more control in the depth of penetration of the skin's surface, allowing an increased degree of precision and safety in treating delicate areas. This procedure could be particularly useful for someone whose skin has been damaged by overexposure to the burning rays of the sun.

I would also seriously consider this procedure for reducing the fine lines around the mouth, which I currently treat with Retin-A. The downtime for recovery from laser resurfacing is approximately two weeks, during which the immediate area may be red and sensitive. For the first few days, the site will be treated with ointment and bandages and must be protected from sunlight. Makeup can be worn after seven to fourteen days.

Thermage Advertised as a nonsurgical face-lift, this newer procedure must be performed by a cosmetic surgeon. Intrigued by this noninvasive approach, I investigated it for myself. The advanced technique uses radio frequency energy to send heat deep into the skin tissues, thereby activating the renewed production of collagen in older skin. Clients experience a brief, intense sensation of heat when the skin is touched by the Thermage instrument, as the collagen in the deep layers of the skin tightens. To protect your skin and make the treatment more comfortable, a cooling spray is delivered before, during, and after each application of the treatment tip. Additionally, as part of pretreatment, a slightly numbing anesthetic cream is usually applied.

The goal is to achieve a tighter, fresher, rejuvenated appearance.

Although the procedure is reputed to involve no downtime, it seems to vary from patient to patient. You may well be red and swollen immediately following it. Thermage claims to:

✓ Tighten the skin all over the face
✓ Lift the eyebrows
✓ Tighten loose skin around the chin, jaw, and neck
✓ Soften the appearance of scarring caused by acne
✓ Soften deep forehead creases and laugh lines

Because I thought the procedure sounded appealing I booked a date to have it done right before a new film project, about six years ago. However, I was forced to cancel, because it was too close to the start of filming. Since then, I've been on the lookout for some conclusive feedback about the safety and effectiveness of Thermage. I know only a few people who have tried it. The first said that she wasn't very impressed. Another said the results were good but not long-lasting. There is no wide-ranging consensus yet on the effectiveness and duration of the improvement. I'm glad now that I didn't go ahead with it. It's amazing what one will consider when the pressure is on to live up to expectations. As you can see, I'm not immune to such impulses!

Oxygen facials   Oxygen facials and products touting oxygen as a skin enhancer are hot right now. The treatment involves a machine that sprays atomized skin treatments, like hyaluronic acid, onto the skin by means of a stream of pressurized oxygen. This is supposed to superhydrate the skin immediately. Oxygen facials are reputed to calm inflammation, treat acne, kill bacteria, and drive antioxidants and vitamins into the skin, making your skin temporarily appear smoother and plumper. Interesting, isn't it?

The only woman I know who has tried oxygen facials did not notice that much difference. But the hype claims it's the ultimate in hydration therapies with instant and long-lasting effects. Celebrities seem to flock to it as a temporary fix, perfect for red-carpet appearances.

As trendy as the oxygen facial may be, there is no hard evidence that it works, and academic experts are skeptical. The lack of clinical evidence has not prevented prominent dermatologists from offering oxygen facials for up to $500 a pop and requiring six weekly treatments, followed by monthly "maintenance" visits. Ouch!

I've heard that a certain major diva has purchased an oxygen facial machine so she can have treatments at home. When the time is right, perhaps it's worth a try. However, at that price, you might want to get a personal recommendation first.

The Lure of Cosmetic Surgery

For many people, cosmetic surgery has become a way of life. They can't wait to regale you with stories of what they've had done. Every Hollywood gathering is rife with exaggerated blow-up lips belonging to people who've become addicted and can't seem to stop. It doesn't hurt to remind oneself that even well-known Hollywood beauties, who have access to so-called A-list surgeons, have ended up destroying the very features that made them famous and have seriously handicapped their careers in the process.

I think we must all applaud those women who have resisted the trend to struggle against the ravages of time, preferring to grow old gracefully, as we used to call it. Their decision is admirable because they accept the visible changes aging brings and seem comfortable in their own skin. Or, perhaps they have done something so slight—like neatening up their chin line—that it looks completely natural. I feel that the proliferation of cosmetic procedures is responsible for a "done look," which is completely out of character and has the stamp of denial.

Starting Younger and Younger

Facial surgery is a serious decision and most definitely has its risks. Even so, the risks involved have failed to dampen consumer enthusiasm. This cavalier attitude is so commonplace that it is attracting younger and younger women into the fold, many of whom are itching to get started. What was once a last resort is now almost as casual as ordering a latte.

There's a popular theory making the rounds that the earlier you start cosmetic procedures the better. I'm not in favor of this at all. Clearly, it sends the wrong message to younger women, unless of course, they have some feature they really can't live with. Rhinoplasty—a reshaping of the nose—and surgery for protruding ears are among the most common reasons for younger people to seek corrective surgery. Peer pressure is a challenge for most young people, and sometimes a reasonable improvement to their physical appearance can help boost self-confidence. But many still-young women are already into mini procedures, for example, the "weekend face-lift." As one article I read states, "The entire industry just feeds into an epidemic of human self-loathing." By the time such a young woman becomes middle-aged, she's at risk of becoming a nip-tuck junkie.

A conceit that has grown into female dogma loudly states, "This is my body, and I can do whatever I want with it!" I don't subscribe to that view. I believe that our life and our body are a gift from our creator. We didn't have any say in the matter. We certainly didn't choose what race, coloring, height, length of limb and features we would be given or what intellect and abilities we would possess. But whatever the raw material we start out with, we will be held accountable for how we treat it, because it has been entrusted to our custody. In other words, we are responsible for our actions, even as they relate to ourselves, because we do most definitely affect other people and the world around us. Whatever you do with God's handiwork, be respectful of the original intent, which in this case means, don't try to look like anyone else.

Your goal when approaching cosmetic surgery should be to improve what you've got, while loving and respecting yourself for who you are.

The Next Best Thing

We are all familiar with the many cosmetic procedures that exist, from face-lifts to eye-lifts, brow-lifts to neck-lifts, to name a few. Information about these and many other options is easy to come by, if not common knowledge. As the demand for altering one's physical appearance has grown, so has the number of newfangled methods that are designed to appeal to those looking for innovative ways to fight Father Time.

After visiting several websites in my research for the latest methods on the scene, I came across a description of the "weekend lift," also called the "thread lift." It is advertised as the equivalent of a new hairdo for an important occasion. I read the description of what one variation of the thread lift entails: a surgeon uses a thin needle to insert barbed sutures under the facial tissue. The procedure can include as many as twenty threads. That was enough for me. Now, doesn't that sound as harmless as a new hairdo? *Not!*

Every year there's a new best thing. The greatest discovery ever! Well, maybe and maybe not. I'm not convinced that we should rush to try every novelty that comes along, while the jury is still out. After all, cosmetic work is always elective and it holds no guarantees. Its risks are high and its remedies limited.

Kinder, Gentler Methods

Luckily, for older women, the cavalry has arrived! Over the past few decades, women have been the beneficiaries of some incredible break-throughs in anti-aging techniques. There are better options for maintaining your appearance than going under the knife. These new innovations are far less drastic and invasive. They started to surface about thirty years ago to great enthusiasm.

An explosion of injectable solutions has changed the face of beauty and become a regular part of its "menu du jour." However, please don't feel compelled to choose one of everything offered, as though you were shopping from a list in the supermarket. That could be a recipe for disaster. The treatments described below have proved to be effective, provided they are administered by a qualified doctor in the field, with appropriate restraint, good taste, and judgment. A personal reference for such a doctor from a friend, family member, or someone else you trust is probably the best way to go about it.

Botox   At the front of the line, Botox injections can boast the ability to impede the progress of wrinkling. Botox is currently one of the most popular anti-aging methods in use. It was approved by the FDA in 2002 and is the brand name for a neurotoxic protein produced by the bacteria *Clostridium botulinum*. When injected into facial muscles, it smoothes out frown lines, forehead creases, and brow furrows by partially paralyzing the muscles underneath. Some people go further and use Botox to lessen crow's-feet and soften thick bands in the neck area.

The downside is that too much Botox can greatly reduce your range of facial expressions, because it blocks muscle contractions. That's scary! If you decide to use it, make sure your doctor understands that you prefer an absolute minimum until you can assess your reaction to this toxin. Remember: botulinum toxins work by temporarily paralyzing some of your facial muscles. Easy does it.

You can always spot overly Botoxed women in restaurants, because they are unable to drink properly. Their numbed lips can't pucker! This embarrassing outcome has happened often enough to make it the brunt of many a late-night comic monologue.

Though many believe that no downtime is involved with Botox, it's unwise not to set aside a period for possible swelling and bruising to subside. Botox has a learning curve. Indeed, anytime you monkey around with Mother Nature, it's best to allow some lead time. She might strike back.

One worrisome trend that has been reported on the news is "Botox on wheels"—basically, minivan clinics that make Botox house calls. There are, apparently, also "Botox parties," the new equivalent of neighborhood Tupperware get-togethers. Both of these unregulated phenomena are clearly risky and likely to be utilizing unlicensed practitioners, who have somehow procured Botox from unofficial sources. Such options, of course, show a reckless disregard for safety and should be avoided.

Injectable dermal fillers Dermal fillers are used to fill in the wrinkles and creases left behind by our daily facial expressions. When the wrinkles are filled by FDA-approved collagens or hyaluronic acid, the signs of aging are temporarily erased, eliminating or delaying the need for surgery. Let's take a brief look at some of them.

The use of collagen as a filler began approximately thirty years ago. Collagen is a natural protein found in bone, cartilage, skin, and tendon that is essential for the strength and elasticity of the skin. The collagen fillers used most by dermatologists are bovine-based, meaning derived from cows. Some patients may be allergic to bovine collagen and should be tested by their doctor prior to facial injections.

Collagen remains the forerunner in a long line of plumping solutions to fill in wrinkles or to augment the lips. The current top brand-name collagen-based fillers, Zyderm and Zyplast, are most frequently used to fill in fine wrinkles and vertical labial folds on either side of the mouth. They are also used to restore the lip border. The procedure involves multiple injections to supplement the natural collagen in your skin. The initial swelling at the injection sites usually fades within a few hours. The fillers will typically need to be refreshed after three to six months.

There are also hyaluronic acid–based fillers, sold under the brand names Restylane, Juvéderm, and Perlane, which can be used in the same manner. All the hyaluronic gel fillers are based on the same kind of acid, but the size of the particles within each differs. Consult your doctor about which particle size is best suited for your treatment. These injections usually last about six months.

Restylane is currently the world's bestselling dermal filler. This hyaluronic acid is reputed to be longer-lasting than collagen. Because of the size of the Restylane particles, some patients experience discomfort at the injection sites with the use of Restylane. You can expect slight redness, swelling, pain, tenderness, itching and/or bruising following Restylane treatment, which could take a few days or more to subside.

CosmoPlast and CosmoDerm fillers are made from highly purified human collagen. These brands last only two to three months.

Any filler that is injected to excess can wind up making you look bloated, like a doughy character from an Austin Powers movie. However, done with finesse, an application of topical anesthetic and nerves of steel, the result can be an effective, noninvasive way to achieve a more youthful appearance.

Necessity Is the Mother of Invention

For a large percentage of women who belong to the boomer and fifty-plus demographic, these less-invasive methods have come just in the nick of time. Both Botox and injectable fillers have been almost as life-altering as the Pill was in the '60s. They have certainly satisfied a growing need. Many women in this age group are more forward thinking and physically fit than the previous generation, and are seeking practical ways to look as good as they feel. Having other alternatives to that old relic, the face-lift, is a welcome relief. Every generation in its time believes it has broken new ground and discovered a brave new world. But is this really the case?

I saw Maureen O'Hara several years ago, up close and personal, and she looked amazing and not done. It was obvious to my eye that she wasn't the subject of some fly-by-night trend. Whatever it was, she looked thirty years younger than she must have been. As far as I can tell, from the days of Claudette Colbert to Cher, women have always managed to "pull it together"—some with a lighter touch and others more boldly. In that regard, things remain pretty much the same.

TMJ Splint— The Anti-aging Effect

Sometimes health-related treatments can have a positive effect on your appearance. The results may be gradual and unexpected, but in the final analysis, time and time again, I've found that health translates into beauty. Case in point: Years ago, I was suffering from migraine-like headaches and visiting a chiropractor, sometimes twice a day. The pain started to spread down my shoulder and across my chest and continue down the entire left side of my body as far as my foot. I even had trouble walking and worried that I might have some dreadful neuromuscular disease. One day my daughter, Tahnee, took one look at me, saw how I was suffering and said, "Mom, you have TMJ! I know a great doctor and he's only two blocks away!"

So I went to see Harold Gelb, D.M.D., the pioneer innovator in the field of TMJ treatment. The cause for my discomfort, Gelb said, was my habit of clenching my jaw and grinding my teeth when under stress. This was an unconscious habit of mine, which over time had worn down my temporo-mandibular joint (TMJ) so that my jaw wasn't adequately supported. It was causing the nerves surrounding that joint to become inflamed and go into spasm, the reason for the radiating pain I was suffering from.

After taking impressions of my bite, Gelb fitted me for a jaw splint, which was like a precisely designed jaw leveler, which he clicked into place. I was instructed to wear this splint while sleeping, exercising, working at the computer, or during any activity, such as long-distance driving, when unconscious tension might be centered in my jaw—a habit of millions of Americans. Within forty-eight hours my pain was relieved, and I have worn a TMJ splint ever since.

Over time I became aware of the anti-aging side effects of this device. By supporting my jaw and keeping it in balance, my splint was also keeping the whole bottom half of my face supported. From my ears down through my chin and jawline, my splint was helping to prevent the skin from drooping. I told Dr. Gelb about this, and he was not surprised. He told me that way back in 1965 he had been interviewed by *Vogue* about using this type of splint. The article was called "New De-wrinkle," and it described the use of the splint as the "world's latest face-lift." In the article Gelb described the TMJ splint as "a plastic fitting over the lower teeth to correct faulty jaw relationship."

As we age, our gums and the bones in our jaw shrink somewhat, causing the skin of the lower face to become a bit slack. By supporting the jaw in its ideal position, the TMJ splint can counteract the aging process, to a greater or lesser degree depending on bone structure. Gelb likes to describe the benefits by saying that "in its simplicity, it's radical." Kinda cool, isn't he? Believe me, I was delighted to hear that there was such a solid history behind what I was now seeing in my bathroom mirror. Hallelujuah! What a wonderful thing!

However, don't go rushing off to get a TMJ splint if you don't need one. This is my personal observation, and I wanted to share it because it's a health-related remedy. Yogis are attuned to many subtle bodily changes, which are the telltale signs of premature aging.

NINE

Hair Hang-Ups!

SUBCONSCIOUSLY, WE RELATE TO OUR HAIR
as the animal, or sexual, side of our nature. Our basic animal instincts
play a role in determining how we deal with this eruption of the beast
within. You could also say that hair is like our own unruly child; it can
interfere with the sanity of daily living, unless we give it our complete
attention and frequent affectionate care.

Scientifically speaking, a strand of hair is just a protein filament
that grows through your skin from a follicle deep under its surface; yet
within it lies all the elements of each person's DNA. A strand of hair
holds many secrets. Even after death, it can be analyzed for traces of
diseases, poisons, drugs, and other data. Hair is a long-term record of
what happens in a person's life.

Fascinating, isn't it? It's not surprising, then, that your hairstyle
can reveal a lot about you all by itself. Through it others will be able to
spot some of your strengths, weaknesses and fears — just by glancing at
your "do."

So many women try to hide behind their hair. When I see actresses
who have two long "curtains" of hair hanging on either side of their face,
I'm always intrigued. As they move, those curtains seem to close
around them. It gives you the feeling that there is something they don't

like about themselves and don't want to show. I've done it myself, in a similar way, believing that if my hair looked good, no one would look too closely at *me*. How you deal with your hair is really a question, I think, of whether you can make friends with the sensual side of your nature and strike a happy medium between letting your hair do its natural thing (perhaps that's what is meant by "letting your hair down") and gently harnessing your untamed follicles into an expression of your personality and style. Hair is an attitude. And like the DNA in its strands, it corresponds to our personal history and reflects it, even as far back as our childhood.

When I was a kid, I wore my hair in bangs and long braids, and then graduated to looped braids. Then it was cut, and I wore it in a flirty ponytail, a style that coincided with my interest in boys. I had a crush on a boy named Larry Isham, who wouldn't give me a tumble. One fateful summer, Mother and I thought it might be a good idea to try something more grown-up, since I was starting my first semester in junior high school. Off we went for my virgin appointment at a hair salon! I was twelve.

At the salon, they cut my hair off to just above the shoulder (gulp!) and then curled it into a bouncy '50s style. It felt strange. With shorter hair, my head felt light and breezy.

I was still getting used to it when I walked through the front door of our home. My dad took one look at me and hit the ceiling. He was furious! He wasted little time before putting my head under the bathroom faucet and soaking it through. The offensive curls went limp. I was thoroughly humiliated. According to my father, only whores and harlots wore their hair loose. Who knew? That's the moment I realized that a hairstyle could have sexual implications.

My Latin father wasn't having any of it. The next day I was back in the salon, and the rest of my hair was cut off, until it was only two inches long. The only option was to comb it back into what was then called a "ducktail." I didn't feel very pretty, but I had no choice. I still don't know what Dad was so worried about; I hadn't even hit puberty yet. Even so, my father was determined to keep me from growing up too soon.

Is it any wonder that one day I would end up a sex symbol? Part of it must have come from a subliminal need to defy him. My father is gone now, God bless him; but what a tangled web of conflicting signals he sent into my young head. I needed a compass to guide me through the contradictions. On the one hand, he was overly strict about things like my hair; but on the other, he reacted positively and noticeably to overtly sexy women, suddenly turning on the charm for them, and showing a side of himself that his family normally didn't see. It was hypocritical, and maddening!

Eventually I got used to my short hair, all the while knowing that it didn't feel like the real me. It was clear that my father didn't like seeing me look like a young woman instead of his little girl. The experience stuck in my memory. I still get nervous just thinking about a haircut. Often, I keep putting it off. Just beneath the surface, I've remained that twelve-year-old for much of my life. It's only in writing down the details of how I evolved that I can recognize it.

The Perfect Haircut

Obviously, hair is a sensitive subject for men and women alike. From presidents and first ladies to supermarket clerks, fussing and fretting over hair remains an ongoing pastime, with mixed results. Nothing is as crucial as the way we *cut* it. Because of this, it's common to arrive at the hairdresser with a tear sheet depicting a model or actress. It's actually a good idea. A photo works better than words for describing what you have in mind. Usually, we start with a reference, wanting to look like so-and-so; anyone, in fact, except ourselves. Women are like chameleons; we crave variety and change. And we're good at it, too.

In the past fifty years, the philosophy about a woman's crowning glory has radically changed. Women no longer aspire to wear hairstyles that are tightly constructed and coiffed within an inch of their life. "Big hair," recycled from the "teased" '60s, remains alive and well today. But now, it's less back-combed and not as full in the crown. In 2010 the style is worn long, loose and slightly wavy, or bone straight.

One version or another of "big hair" in the form of long, flowing locks has been in fashion for a very long time. Another option, which is also a throwback to the '60s, was the very short cut made famous by Twiggy. Providing a nice middle ground is the ever-popular bob, inspired by Louise Brooks in her groundbreaking 1929 film *Pandora's Box*, which made Louise and her bob an instant sensation.

Let me name some great contemporary haircuts that have caught my eye. I like Rihanna's short bob (from 2008), as well as Katie Holmes's and Victoria Beckham's short cuts, but both are second only to Halle Berry's famous Grecian boy cut. Meg Ryan's fabulous short tousled look, by genius haircutter Sally Hershberger, became a new classic in the mid-'90s. When it comes to medium-length hair, I like the styles worn by Kate Moss and Charlize Theron. Both are uncontrived, natural, and versatile. Gwyneth Paltrow's hair always looks good, whether long or short. For longer hair, I also like Jessica Alba, Gisele Bündchen, Jennifer Aniston, and Beyoncé.

Men and women alike live in fear of a bad haircut that will subject them to ridicule and embarrassment. I feel especially sorry for the men because there's no place to hide. Nothing is worse than having your ears sheared so they stick out like a sore thumb. It's humiliating, which may be the reason why the army shaves recruits the moment it gets hold of them. Nothing can cut you down to size quicker than a bad haircut. So if you're thinking about going for super short, like Victoria Beckham, give yourself a little lead time before your next big "doo-dah" event. A week or ten days later, it'll look less clipped.

Once you find a good cutter, keep track of her or him. Always keep an eye peeled for those gifted professionals, because *one* of them is never enough. At some point, you're likely to need a backup, and talented cutters are few and far between. Even with a tear sheet in hand, listen to their advice, so that your haircut can be customized to frame your particular face.

Years ago, I had the luck of finding someone who became my personal go-to guy. His name is Teddy Antolin. I've been relying on "Teds," as I call him, for at least a decade. He's multitalented and is always up on the latest styles. He has done everyone from Sharon Stone to Brooke Shields and Penélope Cruz. I go to him at the Sally Hershberger Salon in Los Angeles, but for special events he comes to my home. He is the real deal and does it all: cuts, styles, colors. We've been working together since the beginning of my wig collection eleven years ago. The cool part is that we collaborate so well that we usually get great results!

When your favorite cutter leaves town, it's not a pretty prospect. I think I'd rather lose a husband! (Just kidding.) A couple of years ago, Teds went on tour with David Bowie for about eighteen months. For me it was sheer torture!

I stopped fretting when Teds recommended another cutter who was right there in Sally's salon and fortunately had seen Teddy and me working together. He was familiar with the layered cut I like to wear, so he did a great job. It was right before a movie role with Burt Reynolds and Charles Durning. In the end, my hair looked great. I can't say as much for the movie. The film needed some expert "cutting" too.

Of course, over a long professional life, I've known a number of star haircutters, but they're not always readily available in an emergency. I'm not speaking of hairstylists, who can make even a bad cut look good. But the truth is that cutting talent is rare. Besides, I hate to be bullied (remember my history), or put at the mercy of a total stranger right before an important event. So I've learned to cut my hair by myself in a pinch. Short hair is relatively easy, but when I first cut my own hair from long to short back in the '80s, it took me a whole week. I did it little by little, each day, gaining confidence as I went. For the back, I used my trusty standing mirror, which I describe in the next chapter on makeup. Look Ma, no hands. It's perfect for the back of your head.

Whether I go to a professional for my cut or do it myself, I make sure to wash and dry my hair *before* I go in, because I prefer to be cut *dry*. Did you know that wet hair is longer than dry hair? That's why, after it's blow-dried, it always looks shorter than you thought it would. I don't like that kind of surprise, and I doubt you do, either. So if you're sensitive to such details and always think "they" cut your hair too short, remember to ask them to cut your hair dry.

Going Gray

Most women I know who are past the age of twenty color their hair because they want to. But for those of us over fifty, covering the encroaching gray is no longer an elective, unless you want to go *au naturel*. There are a valiant few who allow themselves to go salt-and-pepper or completely gray or white and look fabulous. If I had a head of hair like Barbara Bush, I might be persuaded to do so myself. But I don't, and in any case, it's not the right choice for my lifestyle.

I remember when Elizabeth Taylor went salt-and-pepper for *Who's Afraid of Virginia Woolf?* and won an Academy Award for her performance. She has always been a beacon of feminine chutzpah. I respect and admire her. But for the rest of us, when the time comes for that telltale gray to start peeking through, there's a decision to be made.

The first gray hairs seem to appear only here and there and are most visible at the root, so waiting for them to take over your whole head is impractical. That's how I started to notice them. It's not that hard to "have your roots done" professionally, so I didn't think of it as a big deal. But the formula for your roots needs to blend with the rest of your hair color and not show any demarcation. And remember that the hair root is always very slightly darker than the rest of your hair. Striking the right balance takes a little thought and consideration. A good colorist should be aware of this, but it's always best to know the score yourself so you can monitor the process.

Another consideration for women interested in a youthful appearance is that, depending on features, the very severe darker tones tend to look too harsh as one ages. However, using a darkish base color with auburn or mixed highlights can look fabulous! Don't be afraid to try something new. It need not be a drastic change, but adding a few blonde or warm highlights might soften your look and hit just the right note.

Over the course of the seasons, because of the temperature and sunshine or lack thereof, your hair color will change naturally on its own. You might like what happens and want to duplicate that look later. Just be aware and sensitive to these subtle changes, without being obsessive about them. The seasons also determine how fast your hair grows. Even how much exercise you do and your diet have an effect on your hair. When it comes to your halo of hair, there's always something new happening. Never a dull moment.

When Your Own Hair Isn't Enough

It's quite a big deal in expense and time to get the right cut and color. The whole process can be unnerving. But if you're ready for a change in hairstyle or color and want to avoid all the costs and procedures, why not try a wig? As we age, our hair tends to thin. Many women also suffer hair loss as they get older. I've noticed in the past ten years that my own hair is not quite as thick as it once was. Plus, the tricks I relied on previously to beef up the volume are less effective. So on occasion I've taken to augmenting my own tresses with extensions or wigs. In today's world, doesn't everybody? As an actress this is familiar ground for me, as it is for women in fashion and modeling.

More than ever in recent years, even younger women are using wigs, falls, and extensions, just as they did in my generation. Big hair is in style all over again! For those of you who are a bit uncertain about the resources available, the following is for you, especially if you suffer from hair loss or alopecia. It's also for those women who are enthusiastic about fashion and are interested in all the options for fabulous hair.

In case you're wondering, I have worn hair additions of one kind or another for many of my professional appearances over the years. If not a full wig, then a hair extension that fits just behind my own hairline and looks natural and stylish. Besides, since I don't have hot-and-cold running hairdressers at my disposal, it's often much easier to take one of my wigs or falls and drop it off with my stylist. He washes it, conditions it, and styles it for me. Then all I have to do is put it on and anchor it down with a few pins. It's a lot less work for me than using a curling iron on each section, brushing it out, and styling it, hoping it will hold up for an entire event. My own hair is sometimes not very cooperative. I know how to coerce it into any style I want, but it doesn't always stay that way.

Extensions and Falls

I know there's hesitation on the part of some women when they think of wigs. Before I knew better, that was my reaction, too. But like most actresses I've had years of experience with wigs, falls, and extensions during my career. In the '60s we all wore falls, which you attach to the crown of your head and comb your own hair back over to blend in. It's a great tool for adding volume and length. Now, for the past twenty years, influenced by the weave techniques of African-American beauties, hair extensions or weaves have resurfaced as the latest fashion craze.

The first time I tried hair extensions was in the late '80s. I had been wearing shorter hair for almost ten years, but now it was growing out and had reached an awkward stage. I'd heard that the next hot thing was hair extensions, which could help achieve the longer look I wanted. So I asked my makeup and hairstylist, Alfonso Noe, to set the whole thing up for me. An extension stylist came to my hotel room and braided three cornrows into my own hair along the back, about an inch or so apart. Then she sewed three ten-inch-long hair wefts onto these rows with a needle and catgut thread. What a woman won't do.

After Alfonso cut the hair, it looked great—rich and full. But less than an hour later, I started to have the fiercest headache imaginable. My scalp became so sensitive I was ready to crack, and the pain could be traced to those nasty little threads sewn so tightly into the cornrows. I was told that the minibraids and threads tend to loosen up within a few days to a week, but I couldn't wait that long. I wanted those blanking things out! Every nerve ending was on fire. My longtime friend who was present at the time took pity on me. Using my cuticle scissors to avoid cutting my hair off, she carefully snipped through those wicked little threads and put me out of my misery. Even after the wefts were removed, my scalp was sore for a week.

That was the last time I tried that, but thousands of women of all ages still use this method without a problem.

Only a few years later, in 1998, I found a way to beat the system when I started the Raquel Welch Wig Collection, which has everything a girl could possibly need in the way of extensions, falls, or wigs. It includes both real hair and state-of-the-art acrylic fibers. Sometimes even I can't tell the difference. As I mentioned earlier, I have been collaborating with my favorite stylist, Teddy, on the wigs. Once I approve the new styles, Teds and Laurence, the style consultant at HairUWear, work closely with me to cut and shape the wig patterns, right on my head. That's how those styles come to life. We recently finished working on the new spring collection for 2010, which promises to be our most popular collection yet.

Wigs to the Rescue

The first time I ever wore a wig was for the movie *Fantastic Voyage* (1964). My role was to play a marine biologist, of all things. Can you picture it? I couldn't . . .

The director, Richard Fleischer, and studio head, Dick Zanuck, decided that I should cut my hair for the role. I agreed that shorter hair would be more appropriate for the character but didn't really want to sacrifice my long tresses. The part of the comely scientist I was about to play amounted to little more than eye candy, in a team of male researchers making a landmark voyage through the human bloodstream. It was an A-list movie, but my part wasn't worth the haircut. When they told me the plot, I was pretty sure that my minor presence in this sci-fi extravaganza wouldn't get much notice.

To my relief, they let me wear a short-hair wig for the role. To do it, I wrapped my long hair closely to my head and pinned it. Over that I put on a close-fitting stocking cap called a wig cap. It made the placement of a short brunette wig secure.

I used to take the thing off at lunch because it was so hot. Innovations in wig technology have changed a lot since then; today's wigs allow the scalp to breathe. Still, back then it was great to wear a wig that made it possible for me to look right for the role but saved me from having to cut off my long hair. It was the first of many movies for which wigs would come to the rescue.

The famous sci-fi epic, *One Million Years B.C.* offered a completely different hair challenge. I played Loana, Queen of the Shell People, and producer Michael Carreras had his heart set on a blonde. Yes, you heard right. She was the good girl. (We know that *because* she's a blonde.) There was also a not-so-good girl, the Queen of the Rock People. She had to have black hair. When we had our famous girl fight, it would be good against evil . . . blonde against brunette. I can't even think about it without cracking up! But I was in no position to argue.

To accomplish my transformation, I was subjected to a truly bad bleach job, which turned my hair bright orange. Clumps of my once virgin hair broke right off and fell to the floor. What the hell? I was unaware that such horror stories were commonplace in the movies.

There is, for example, the well-known story of Jean Harlow, the first platinum blonde. Rumor has it that they used a mixture of Ivory Snow soap and bleach on her head several times a week, to achieve that platinum blonde look. It would seem that a concoction as toxic as this would be dangerous. I guess they did it so often because they didn't want her darker roots to show.

Sadly, somehow Jean got uremic poisoning, though no one could figure out in time what caused it. I don't know what caused Harlow's uremic poisoning, but I do know that anything chemical you put on your scalp, including detergent mixed with bleach, if applied frequently enough, can be toxic. Apparently, much of what is put on your scalp is easily absorbed through the pores and enters your bloodstream.

I myself became wary of going through such a drastic color change, for the role of Loana. In a futile half-measure, I would only allow them to bleach the front half of my hair. I emerged from the process with two-toned hair, the colors divided from ear to ear across the center of my head. The front was orange and broken, while the back was still my own natural brunette color. What a predicament.

In the wake of this debacle, I ended up wearing a custom-made blonde fall rather than risking the possibility of more bleach damage to the rest of my long, dark hair. The fall fit about two inches back from my natural hairline, so that it covered three quarters of my head, but when we were shooting outdoors and the wind blew, you could only see my own hairline around my face. Fortunately, by the time filming began, my hair had lost its offensive orange glow and the fall was an exact match. Nobody guessed it wasn't my own. These two experiences were an eye opener and right in sync with the '60s trend toward big hair! That was when I joined a long list of young actresses of the day who almost without exception wore wigs or hairpieces for various roles.

Even today, my own hair is still quite serviceable and works fine for day-to-day activities. But when I want to pull out the stops and look fabulous, I often prefer to augment my natural resources with either extensions, a fall or, in some cases, a full wig. Sometimes I choose a hairpiece made from 100 percent human hair, but other times I put on a fall made from the new synthetic fibers. In fact, I'm wearing a synthetic wig on the cover of this book. The latest technology is so amazing that you can't tell whether it's human hair or not.

Great Lengths

Although there is an unspoken rule that women of a certain age should not wear their hair long, I have enjoyed wearing mine that way for the past several years. I've also taken to wearing individual hair extensions. Mine are made by Great Lengths for HairUWear, the company that manufactures and distributes my wig collection.

A recent breakthrough in the creation of these 100 percent human-hair extensions has made it possible to add length, volume, or both without compromising the integrity of the natural strands. The extensions now come with a synthetic protein-based bond attached to the root end of each small section of hair. The section is molded to your own hair near the root with the use of a bonding tool. That is why I prefer using Great Lengths. Their extensions have the best bonding, whereas others use glue or wax, which are less effective. If you try this, make sure that a specialist in the field does the application. The process takes no longer than a usual hair appointment.

Heat-Friendly Fibers

After more than a decade of experience with wigs, I've learned that synthetic hair has several advantages. It holds its shape and shine better than real hair. You don't have to curl or style it each time you wear it. It's low-maintenance, travels well, and just needs to be hung upside down on a hanger at night (I use a jumbo safety pin). When the time is right, you can pop it on and style it as you desire with a comb or your fingertips, and then you're ready to go.

The one drawback was that, until recently, especially with longer styles, you couldn't curl, flatiron, or blow-dry synthetic hair. Now you can have that versatility. *News flash! There are new cutting-edge synthetic fibers that are heat friendly and can be curled and waved just like real hair!* Isn't that phenomenal?

The Three Musketeers

Many women who aspire to fabulous hair favor wearing a custom-made wig from 100 percent human hair. I understand that preference but it's quite a complicated process. So I'd like to share an experience I had with my first custom-made, real-hair wig for my role in the film of the Alexandre Dumas classic *The Three Musketeers*. I needed special wigs to achieve the sixteenth-century hairstyles designed for my character, Constance Bonacieux, mistress to the queen. Faye Dunaway and Geraldine Chaplin also wore these gorgeous custom-made wigs, which were manufactured from virgin (meaning not chemically processed) European hair. All three wigs had been made in London and were said to be "very dear." That's the British expression for *expensive*.

I discovered that custom-made real-hair wigs with lace fronts can be time consuming and far from a quick fix. A customized lace front is made from very, very fine hand-knotted lace that must be shaped to your head. To fashion this wig cap, a piece of pliable plastic (like Saran Wrap) is stretched over the skull and strips of cellophane tape are used to secure it very snugly to the exact configuration of your head, leaving space around the ears. There's a very precise art to this taping, which creates the exact fit for the base of your wig. The method for weaving these strips of tape together is very painstaking.

Once this helmet is in place on your head, they trace along your natural hairline with a marker to delineate the way your hair frames your face. Using this pattern, they hand-make the lace from silk, tinting it to match the exact skin tone of your face. Once the hair is knotted into the cap, your hairline will not be visible underneath the finished wig.

In case you're wondering, your own hair is always tucked up underneath the wig, inside the cap. You pin it around and back and secure it with a stocking cap, which holds everything in place.

In real life, as opposed to films, the crucial point is how your wig addresses your hairline. With a custom-made wig, the hair around the face has to be knotted in a forward direction and some of it must come out underneath the edge of the wig as it fits around the face and neck. This camouflages where the wig ends and your hairline begins. A good wig, of course, has to be crafted to simulate hair growing out of your own head.

Even some men wear custom-made, real-hair wigs. I worked with a major male star who had a spectacular hairpiece covering the top of his head. In fact, he had a couple of hairpieces, one for wearing and one in the wings being groomed. He traveled with his own hair guy, who took care of these pieces, which were British-made. The hair was brilliantly knotted around his face, and the hairpiece was undetectable. It was also super short.

Whatever the wig style, only the finest wig makers are qualified to practice this ancient art. This is why good wigs cost an arm and a leg, meaning, many thousands of dollars. Most commercial wigs are made with either synthetic or real hair until recently and address the hairline issue with bangs or a light fringe. I pull about an inch of my own hair out from under my wig and around the face, then comb it into a partic-ular style. I usually curl it slightly from the root so it doesn't lie flat. This helps achieve a natural look, and usually, any slight difference in color is indiscernible.

Women should understand that custom-made wigs are very high maintenance and need to be handled by a professional. They may be worth the investment if you'll be wearing one every day because of per-manent hair loss caused by a disease like alopecia, or just by aging. But if you're someone who is suffering from temporary hair loss due to the complications of illness, including chemotherapy, or you're only inter-ested in wig products as a beauty or fashion accessory, then you are probably better off with a much less expensive wig from a reputable commercial source. For example, the wigs in my collection, both those that are 100 percent human hair and those that are synthetic, are priced at a fraction of the cost of custom-made wigs. And this season we offer cutting-edge new lace front construction.

I wore a beautiful short reddish wig from my own collection (in Glazed Cinnamon) on *Larry King Live* a couple of years ago. Only days later, I was back on the set of the PBS miniseries *American Family* with my own medium-length, soft-brown hair. I've also worn various kinds of hair additions on many talk-show appearances and on film for acting roles since 1998. I'm lucky to have access to all the wigs in my collection. The way I look at it, with the aid of a wig, I have more versatility in my life, and so can you!

A Morale Boost

I'm happy to say that, for the past five years, thousands of my wigs have found their way throughout the country into the lives of women suffering from cancer-related hair loss. Seeing how wigs have helped the morale and self-confidence of these women has been one of the most satisfying and rewarding experiences of my life.

Starting with my first association in 1975 with the American Cancer Society as national spokesperson, I have wanted to find a significant way to help those suffering from this horrible disease. Then, almost five years ago, when my cousin was diagnosed with cancer, she asked me to recommend a wig for her from my collection. It dawned on me that here was something seemingly simple that clearly had the potential to touch her life in an enormous way. Although previously depressed about losing her hair, she soon became thrilled at how attractive she looked in a wig and couldn't wait to show her friends! Her reaction made me realize how devastating it is for a woman to watch her hair fall out. In fact, it has become common knowledge at cancer treatment centers across the country that looking good definitely boosts patient morale, which is vitally important to the recovery and the healing process. The same is the case for those suffering from alopecia.

I still cherish the memory of one very pretty nineteen-year-old who had become almost completely bald from chemotherapy. I was struck by how hard it must be for this young girl, who was a Katherine Heigl look-alike, to face herself in the mirror each day. She asked me for a long blonde wig, smooth and flowing. The look on her face when we slipped this wig onto her head was priceless. The style was a replica of her own hair before she had been diagnosed with cancer. In an instant, she looked as gorgeous as she ever had, and her smile was all the proof I needed.

There were also a number of mature women who needed wigs for patchy baldness, which was obviously a source of embarrassment for them. No matter what the balding pattern, there were a variety of wigs to provide solutions. With a team of volunteers, I worked to select the colors and styles for each of these women. A hairstylist then fit and trimmed each wig to complement individual faces. The ladies were delighted that putting on a wig could be so uplifting and commented on how lightweight and airy the wigs felt on their heads. They, too, couldn't wait to model their new look for family and friends.

I was deeply moved again when I read their thank-you notes. In all honesty, I was the one who owed them a debt of thanks, for letting me share their experience. I have kept many of their notes as souvenirs of what real courage and optimism looks like. Like the soldiers I met in Vietnam so many years ago in 1967, those women fighting off disease left me with a lasting reminder of the better side of the human spirit.

TEN

Makeup

MY GOAL FROM AN EARLY AGE WAS TO BE
an actress, so I've always been into makeup. After I started putting on
plays in my garage and selling tickets to the neighbors, my mother got
the hint and enrolled me, at the ripe old age of seven, in the Old Globe
Junior Theatre in Balboa Park, San Diego. Every summer for years,
I took the bus to the actors workshop for kids, where we were assigned roles in different plays and they taught us how to apply stage
makeup to become different characters. For me, this was beyond
exciting!

I discovered that, in the legitimate theater, actors were traditionally called upon to do their own makeup. It was considered a part of *getting into character*. So I threw myself enthusiastically into practicing the
technique of highlighting and shadowing to change my appearance. I
was fascinated by the idea of "painting" on the three-dimensional canvas of my own face and watching the transformation take place. And I
was good at it. I felt as if I could transform myself into a surprisingly
wide range of characters, from an old crone of a witch, warts and all,
to a radiant young beauty like Juliet. Since then, rightly or wrongly, I
have always equated being a woman with being an actress. It's not a

new concept. As Shakespeare famously wrote in *As You Like It*, "All the world's a stage / And all the men and women merely players."

The idea that I could be self-sufficient when it came to inventing my identity—that I could create my own look and change it at will—made a lasting impression on me. It stuck with me over the years and led me into some real flights of fancy along the way. In the '60s, I was one of many who wore more than one pair of false eyelashes at a time, with pale lipstick and tons of hair. It was great fun and as trendy and rebellious as the period in which it was fashionable. Back then, I was caught up in the moment. After all, I was living and working in fabulous Swingin' London!

There were, of course, times when I did tone things down for special occasions, like meeting Queen Elizabeth at the Royal Command Performance for *Casino Royale*. I also had to adapt my look to accommodate films like *The Three Musketeers* and its sequel, which were sixteenth-century period pieces, and for the '20s flapper film *The Wild Party*, or various westerns. But to this day, I still look on my makeup call as part of getting into character. To some extent, it's the same thing that millions of other women do every day of their lives. Women are always "getting into character." Isn't every one of us an actress, with many roles to play?

Star Treatment?

My first film experience found me waiting my turn in the 20th Century Fox makeup department. So many glorious stars had sat in those same makeup chairs. It was 1964, and one of the contract makeup artists at Fox had been assigned to me for the movie *Fantastic Voyage*. I sat there feeling thrilled about my new contract, but even more about what I imagined I was about to experience: a fabulous Hollywood makeover! I was so eager to be sent through that legendary Hollywood star-making machine. The reality, however, was something quite different.

Without much ceremony or even any careful analysis, a makeup artist arrived and briefly introduced himself. Without any further ado, he tipped me back in the chair and began applying makeup at the speed of light, as though someone were holding a stopwatch. He was finished with me (and I with him), before I could blink: *bing, bang, boom!*

Clearly, he wasn't doing *my* face, but a stock face he had done a million times before. He finished by dusting me with enough powder to set my face for the next century, then swiveled me around in the chair to have a look in the mirror.

I didn't recognize myself! Who in hell was that staring back at me? I looked painted, powdered, and pathetic. I was deeply disappointed. It had suddenly become obvious that the star-making days I'd heard so much about were long gone. Evidently, they had disappeared with the death of Marilyn Monroe, who'd been contracted to this very same studio. I was going to have to fend for myself.

My reaction to this predicament was to jump into my Spitfire, drive like crazy all the way home, wash my face clean, and start from scratch. Even then, I knew my face like Einstein knew physics. It's something I think every actress knows. I also knew exactly what I wanted to look like for this role. I made it back to the set for shooting just in the nick of time, and no one said a word. But before the day was over, it turned out I was in hot water, and I got called onto the carpet at the front office.

"Just who the hell do you think you are?" demanded Dick Zanuck, the head of the studio.

All I could muster was, "I didn't like the way he made me look."

"So," he countered, "you think you know more than the experts?"

"No, but I want to look like myself, and I think I'm the best expert on that subject."

He stared at me, perplexed, then shrugged and seemed to accept my reasoning. "I like your spirit, kid," he said. It broke the ice and we became friends.

The makeup artist who did me that first day never came near me again. He handed me a powder puff and told me I was on my own and I have been ever since. Every day, I brought my own paint box, with all my brushes and pencils. It sure came in handy. No newcomer gets an exclusive makeup artist assigned to her before she becomes a breakthrough star. Quite often, there's no one around when you need 'em.

Of course, today I'm very grateful for the many talented makeup artists who've helped me look my best on film over the years. They collaborated with me on each role I played. They have shared their secrets, taught me about lighting, and watched over me on camera as no one else could. Many of them remain my close pals. One of my favorites was the late British makeup genius John O'Gorman. He really refined my look from "done" into natural beauty for the movie *Hannie Caulder*. For women in film, there was none better, with the exception of the Italian makeup artists, who are in a class of their own.

For both film and commercial photography sessions, I still work with talented artists whose contribution is invaluable. Terri Apanasewicz, Francesca Tolot, Joanne Gair, and Charlotte Tilbury are all exceptional. They have humored me and worked with me to invent different looks. They've added refinements, blended out my errors, and steered me away from dated choices. I'm proud to say that, in the process, I did become somewhat of an expert and I'm happy to pass along some of the tricks of the trade.

Accentuate the Positive— Eliminate the Negative

Over the years I've adapted the principles of using highlight and shadow that I learned back in my junior-theater days for use in daily life. The practice is called *corrective makeup* in the trade. It's a technique that can enhance, and even reshape, your features. You can correct and soften those flaws that you're least fond of, alter the appearance of your bone structure, and diminish the signs of aging. Used in this way, makeup can enable you to put your best face forward.

The texture of the makeup you use for highlighting and shadowing should be more like pan-stick than liquid makeup. This allows you to control its placement. *For highlighting, use a color slightly lighter than your foundation; and for shadowing, use one that's slightly darker.* If you choose colors and tones according to these principles, they will be subtly effective but undetectable when blended.

You can use highlights and shadows to narrow and shorten your nose, and to accentuate your cheekbones or play them down. You can shadow your brow bone to open up your eyes and make them seem bigger. You can downplay a protruding forehead. You can reshape your mouth and make your lips look fuller. Using shadowing, you can define your chin line. The following are a few tips for using highlights and shadows.

Redefine your nose.   You can use a highlighter down the bridge of your nose and a darker color on the sides to make your nose appear narrower. If you want your nose to seem shorter as well, put a touch of shadow at the tip. Be sure to blend.

I know a very famous beauty whose nose has a deep indentation at the middle of the bridge, which makes it look quite flat. This isn't noticeable in photos because her makeup artist cleverly paints a shiny substance into the flat part of the nose, which raises and hides the indentation. He follows up by blending the shine down the whole length of the nose to make the entire bridge look higher. And, of course, he shadows the sides with a slightly darker base, to make the nose look narrower. The effect is gorgeous.

Change the look of your cheekbones.   By experimenting with highlights and shadows, you can modify or accentuate the shape of any feature, including cheekbones. Applying a shadow blusher just under the cheekbone will emphasize the hollow and accent the structure of the whole face. I prefer *not* to highlight my cheekbones, because they are already quite prominent—they catch enough light. But most women can improve their face by brushing the top of the cheekbone with a high-sheen powder. Most often, I use a mustard-colored blusher to de-emphasize my cheekbones. You should always go by what is right for your specific features.

Emphasize your chin line.   You can also use shadow blush to carefully accentuate your chin line. If you want to correct your chin line by giving it more definition, try the following: Looking at your reflection from the side, dab your shadow blush with a sponge. Then run the sponge along your jawline to create the ideal shape. Blend it down under the chin, if needed. If this looks too strong, tone it down by putting a touch of foundation on your sponge. Finish with translucent powder. Be sure to check your face from all angles when using this technique.

For all these sculpting techniques, I encourage you to seek the advice of a makeup artist, who can give you a practical demonstration. There are quite a few good ones in most department and beauty supply stores, such as Sephora, and especially in the MAC cosmetic boutiques, where the makeup artists are always excellent pros. I love the colors of MAC's shadows and pencils. They also have wonderful brushes and a modulated spectrum of lip colors.

Do It Yourself

Before you start to apply your makeup, it's important that you establish your own "get-ready" space, or portable makeup station. I find this indispensable. Who needs the frustration of leaning over a bathroom sink, or worse, balancing a handheld mirror in one hand while applying eyeliner with the other? It gets old fast. Here are some simple ways to solve the problem by creating your own mini makeup station.

Your mirror   I have a wonderful adjustable standing mirror, which I position in front of my makeup table or bathroom sink. It's about five and a half feet tall so I can move it around until I find a good place for it. It stands on a base with a telescoping pole that can be adjusted to various heights. The mirror has a magnifying side and also a regular side, both of which can be swiveled into position easily. That way, I get two perspectives. I find it indispensable and don't know what I'd do without it. I can do the close work first with the magnifying side and then flip to the other side to check the overall effect.

For daytime occasions, I like to do my face in daylight near a window. I've been using my adjustable mirror since the mid-'70s for such occasions. I also use it for evenings because it comes in handy for doing the close work. Finally, I can break it down for travel and pack it in my suitcase.

Because I'm spoiled, for evening I have a *lighted makeup mirror* that is surrounded by frosted white bulbs on a rheostat, so that I can adjust the brightness. Another option would be to purchase a portable lighted makeup mirror. Some of them even have settings for day and evening and can be set on a table in front of which you can sit comfortably to do your face. If the mirror is too low, try using a couple of telephone directories to raise it to face height. There are also wall-mounted mirrors that can be helpful.

Your lighting Obviously, you always need to see clearly when you apply your makeup. Doing your face in bad light can result in sometimes clownish effects. I get a lot of compliments on my makeup, which I attribute to the fact that I do my face in good light. For everyday purposes, you may not have a facility like a star dressing room, but you can improvise a homemade solution.

If you own an adjustable standing mirror, as described above, or can acquire one (available at www.imperialmirror.com), find some source of good balanced natural light that doesn't cast deep shadows on your face. Set up a mirror and a chair there during the day. Make sure the light is indirect, not hitting you smack in the face. If this is unavoidable, pull sheer curtains or shades over the window or back your chair away from the light source. Once you've settled on a good, comfortable place to do your face, you'll need your makeup and tools close by—and they'll need to be organized.

Organizing your makeup   I always keep my makeup, brushes, and other tools in a *Lucite cosmetics tray* that has brush and pencil holders and/or a drawer divider. This gives me a single contained place to lay out my tools for easy access. It also allows me the equivalent of a *portable makeup tray*. I can easily move my stuff around from one room to another if needed. Try it!

I got the idea from working as an actress on movie sets. For my early films, I carried a small painter's watercolor box around with me. I could pack it with my essential supplies and take it anywhere. I have brought it onto airplanes in my flight bag and into airport lounges for a touch-up. I have used it in hotel rooms and moved it from window to bathroom. It accompanied me on photo shoots, into trailer dressing rooms, and on all my film sets. Once, I took it aboard a small boat while we were filming on the Côte d'Azur, because no makeup artist could get to me there.

There are countless occasions on a movie set when running back and forth every time you need something isn't very efficient. Having my box stashed nearby was a great timesaver. In fact, I was rarely without my trusty little kit. I mounted a mirror on the wooden paint palette kept inside it. That way, I was ready for anything . . . even the paparazzi.

Your Products and Tools

What follows is a list of items I consider essential.

An effective moisturizer   It should have at least 15 SPF protection, or a tinted moisturizer that can correct your coloring under a sheer foundation. They come in various shades, from pale green to counteract redness to peachy tones to bring warmth to sallow skin.

A foundation base   Choose from liquid, pan-stick, creamy base, or mineral-powder foundations. It depends on personal taste and what works best on your skin. In my teens, I started out using a creamy liquid and then graduated to Max Factor Pan-Stik in the Sun Tone shade. I've also used bronzing gels.

It's interesting to try different products, so I've experimented with nearly everything out there, for different purposes. Most recently, I've been working with two foundations: a pan-stick base color and a cream foundation of lighter texture for corrections. Between the two, I get good results.

Top-quality sponges   Your sponges should be tightly meshed, without big holes, for a smooth application. They come in five-by-five-inch blocks precut into perfect wedges for best handling and effect. Test for softness and pliability.

Concealer   I only use concealer, which is thicker in texture than foundation base, for trouble spots, such as darkness under the eyes and other flaws. The color should be slightly lighter than your foundation, *but not a stark white*. Otherwise, you'll end up with raccoon eyes, so don't go for a big contrast. Concealers come in cover sticks, in small jars, in tubes, or in wands, like YSL's Hi-Lite Brush. The consistency varies but should always cover easily and then disappear. I often use Ben Nye Medium/Tattoo Cover NP 4.

Try using a *concealer brush* to apply concealer (or highlighter) in specific areas. It's a flat, smallish, spatula-shaped brush. It's the best way to apply the product under the eye, on blemishes, or in the nasal labial folds extending from either side of your nose to the corners of your mouth. You can also use this brush for countless other corrections, such as applying a slightly lighter shade of foundation around the nostrils, just inside them, and around the mouth area, especially near the corners of the mouth. It's also handy for applying MAC's Prep + Prime base to your eyelids before applying eye shadow.

Eyeliner   You'll need at least two shades of eyeliner, one softer shade, such as a taupe, for day, and one darker tone for evening, such as charcoal. You have a choice of pencil, liquid, or cake. I use taupe by MAC under the eye and a black cake liner next to my upper lashes and sweeping up and out at the sides. Q-tips are good for smudging and blending, if needed. I always powder over the bottom liner with a small brush, so that the color doesn't smudge or transfer to other places around the eyes.

Eye shadow   I suggest using at least three colors. Choose a light tone, a medium tone, and a dark tone of your favorite color. This allows you to blend and give dimension to the color. If you apply it with an eye-shadow stick or pencil, blend thoroughly with a brush and dust with powder.

To get the best effect from your eye shadow, I suggest three brushes for the eyes: (1) *an eye-lining brush*; (2) *a second "unfluffy" brush with softly graduated tip* to give dimension to your eye shadow without leaving a hard line; and (3) *a small brush with a rounded, fluffy shape*, which can be used to blend and lightly dust shade on shade, over your base shadow.

The "unfluffy" brush is ideal for reshaping the ridge above the eye with dry shadow; this has the corrective effect of making your eyes look bigger, so you'll want the placement to be more controlled. The brush with the rounded, fluffy shape is versatile and can also be used for dusting a neutral color, like MAC's Wedge, over the entire lid, which pulls the whole eye together.

For the eyebrows   A self-sharpening eyebrow pencil is best. Maybelline makes one. Otherwise, have a *double sharpener* ready. It has a hole for large pencils and one for smaller pencils. You can't do a decent job on your eyebrows without a sharpened pencil. You should also find a small wedged brush for applying cake brow filler.

Lip moisturizer   Get one that works well under makeup. Don't laugh, but I use Bag Balm, which is what dairy farmers use on cow udders when milking. I know it's weird, but it works. My daughter Tahnee told me about it when she was modeling.

Lip brush and lipstick Retractable brushes are best, because the tip must be protected. In general, *the darker the lipstick color, the older it makes you look*. Younger girls with certain shades of blonde hair can sometimes get away with reds, but as a rule, stay with soft colors such as peach, coral, pink, or just a tinted lip gloss. These are far more inviting. In my experience, most men don't like intense lipstick colors in person-to-person encounters. Believe it or not, when they are sitting across the table from you, they want to see natural-looking lips, not a slash of color. So stay clear of the Joker look. Marilyn Monroe and Elizabeth Taylor both wore red lipstick to stunning effect, so if you look like either one, then go ahead and rock that red! Being an olive-skinned girl, I seldom go there.

For several film roles, I needed a natural nude look on the lips. To achieve that effect without losing the shape and delicate natural color of the lips, I used MAC's Vegas Volt, a more intense lip color, as a base to stain my lips, but blotted it *waaay* down. Next, I tapped a smidgen of base over it and added a touch of lip balm. It gave me a lovely, natural, but juicy color. To correct the shape of my mouth, I lined my lips with a nude color like MAC's Spice mixed with Mochaberry Automatic Lip Liner, blending the liner very carefully to make sure there was no hard edge. After that, I blotted the edge with a folded-flat facial tissue. Finally, I dusted just the lip edge with a hint of powder, making it invisible to the eye. It worked.

Blushers Most people like compact blushers. They are quite easy to use. These, of course, are best applied with a large, fluffy brush. I apply blusher right over my unpowdered foundation and blend it with my base sponge. (See more about blush application under "My Step-by-Step Routine.")

Darker cake blushers are known as *contouring blushers*. Use them for shadowing in the hollows of the cheeks and along the chin line. They can be used anywhere you want to diminish a feature like a prominent forehead or jaw, or even on the very tip of your nose to make it look shorter, as described earlier.

Powder   In my opinion, loose translucent powder works the best. It's more refined and can be applied sparingly with a powder brush. I use a large, fluffy white brush to dust my forehead and lower cheeks. I don't pile powder on my cheeks or around my eyes. For these areas, I use a medium-size barrel brush. And I only tap it on the places that pop with shine. I find that as you get older, *the more powder you apply over fine lines, the more you will accentuate them.*

My Step-by-Step Routine

Since each of us is unique, I will not presume to tell you exactly how to do your face. Makeup is an important statement of your own personal style and should be developed over time on your own. But since we all learn from one another, here's how I make up my own face, along with a few suggestions and explanations of the techniques I use.

Moisturizer   Before I begin making up, I apply moisturizer to my face and neck and give it a chance to sink in. I use one that works under makeup, not a thick, heavy night cream. If your skin is oily, perhaps you won't need one. In that case, just apply toner instead, as there is already some moisturizer in most makeup. There are also balancing solutions on the market that can treat oily skin. If a film of moisture remains on the surface of your face after you've applied your moisturizer, toner, or balancing solutions, blot lightly with a single flat facial tissue.

Eye drops   I use eye drops every morning after I brush my teeth. I think they are a great beauty treatment, and my eyes love them. They help soothe away dryness and irritation from overheated rooms or tiredness. I use the kind that takes the red out, to clear away the "road maps" in my eyes. But if your eyes are very sensitive, I recommend you consult a doctor first.

Eyes   I usually do my eyes next, so that I won't disturb my foundation later. Mascara, eye shadow, and other products can interfere with
a flawless overall finish.

First I curl my lashes with a *lash curler* and dust them with a little
bit of powder before applying mascara; it makes them thicker. Repeat
the process, if you like. I use a waterproof mascara in black. Blondes
might prefer dark brown.

Next I apply *pencil liner* under the eye, next to the lashes. For a
more dramatic effect, I sometimes extend the line past the outer corner,
subtly slanting up — not down. I smudge this with a Q-tip and powder
it with a small powder brush (square tip, ⅛-inch wide). It helps to blend
and set the liner. I also line the upper lid with a pencil, then powder it
and finish with a thin liquid liner along the upper lash.

Before I add my eye shadow, I apply a *primer*. My favorite is Prep +
Prime by MAC. Apply it to the top eyelids. It helps the shadow go on
smoothly and sets it.

For *eye shadow*, I have three favorite colors that work together: Satin
Taupe, a neutral color, for day; Fake, a darker "midnight" tone, for a dramatic smokey eye; and third, Aria, a medium-dark shade that fits perfectly between the other two — all three colors by MAC. This gives me
lots of options. The darker color adds more definition and glamour for
evenings and red-carpet events. If you're brave enough, you can also incorporate a touch of color shadow, like blue, green, or mauve, over the
base shadow. When I'm in the mood, I add an extra dash of eye-shadow
color — blue or mauve or burgundy — under the lower lash, just over the
liner, creating a hint of color that softens the whole look. Don't forget
to blend.

For evenings, you can try a whisper of golden or silvery shimmer.
Brush it lightly on the brow bone over your taupe or smoky shadow,
using a wedge-shaped brush. You might also want to add shimmer with
a small brush under your lower lash and over your liner. If you don't
have one, use a Q-tip and blend.

For more allure, try sweeping your eye shadow outward toward the temples. Or, if you want to subdue the final effect, dust your shadow with a touch of face powder to bring it down a notch.

Foundation   A foundation color must blend with your skin tone and enhance it. Try some on the inside of your wrist first as a test. The skin on your face is usually lighter than the rest of your body. It's supposed to be. Even if you're very tan, your face and neck should be a few shades lighter than the rest of you.

I apply my foundation with a light touch, making sure to get coverage where it's needed. Sometimes it's helpful to add a dab of moisturizer to the sponge. As I mentioned, you can use a tinted moisturizer first and then apply a light foundation over it.

Remember: When you apply foundation, everything must be blended. No harsh lines, and don't stop at the chin. Blend down the neck. I use a small sponge or my fingertips. Check your chin line from the side with a hand mirror.

Highlighting   For highlighting, select a shade slightly lighter than your base, but one that also blends with your foundation color and texture. You can use your highlighting to camouflage signs of aging. Apply it to the delicate area under the eyes and blend outward all the way past the corner of the eyes, above the cheekbones. It should be a light consistency, not too heavy, or it will accentuate wrinkles. Apply also around the nostrils and along both labial folds, from your nose to the corners of your mouth, if needed. Blend perfectly with your fingertips.

I always wait until later in the process to powder the area under my eyes. Usually some tiny slivers of excess makeup will form in fine lines around the eyes or other areas. Tap them lightly with a fingertip to smooth them away, but don't drag. Powder lightly with your fluffy barrel powder brush. Again, do not drag.

Because I find my cheekbones are too prominent, I like to diminish them a little with a Sun Tone base, which I apply to my cheekbones to soften them a bit. I also sharpen my jawline with shadow. This focuses the attention on the inverted triangle formed by the eyes, nose and lips. The visual focus is supposed to be on this part of the face. However, you can adjust your own triangle-zone focus up or down to complement your features.

Think about where the best focus is for your face. Because I have a strong jaw, I like the focus raised a little. I accentuate my bone structure from the corner edge of my mouth upward, as far out as the ends of my eyebrows. But I don't exaggerate, because it shouldn't be obvious. It takes a very light touch.

Blusher   I like peachy colors to go with my skin tone. Depending on the occasion, I like to apply a cream blusher very gingerly with a sponge. I place it in a diagonal area fanning out from the cheek apple to the temple. I blend it with my base sponge so it doesn't look like rouge. Blush should look like the glow of health, not like makeup. I barely powder this area, preferring a soft glow. After this, I apply a touch of Sunset cake blusher by Make Up For Ever to my cheeks, temples, forehead, chin tip, and jawline. When I'm tanned, I use some goldenrod-colored blusher over the cheeks, forehead, and jaw, to give a sun-kissed glow. I learned this years ago from an African-American model I worked with, and I've found that it's very effective on olive skin, too.

Because I have a strong jaw, I use a tan blusher to shade the area between my jawline and the blusher on my cheekbones.

Powder   Most women use too much powder. For my own, non-oily skin, I try to ensure that my makeup has a dewy, natural glow. My technique for applying any kind of loose powder, whether translucent or colored like blusher, is to dip my brush into the product and then tap the handle with my finger to get rid of the excess before lightly dusting my face.

You can easily add more powder if needed, but it's harder to remove it. If you do go overboard, dab a clean sponge with moisturizer and swipe it across the back of your hand. Then dab it lightly across the overly powdered areas. That should lift the dry, parched look. After powdering you can also try a sprinkling of rosewater on a damp piece of cotton to add a natural sheen.

Cheekbones To emphasize my bone structure, I shadow very lightly under my cheekbones with a dark coppery base color. Easy does it. You can also do this with dry contour blushers. Use a fluffy-tipped brush.

Eyebrows Using a well-sharpened pencil, lightly sketch in individual hairs to fill in the places where your eyebrows are thinner. Keep your pencil strokes in a diagonal slant to match the direction of your natural eyebrow hairs. Painted-on brows look too artificial. Use a pencil half a shade lighter than your color as well as a clean brow brush to soften the pencil strokes. Powder away the shine.

Eyelashes False eyelashes are a whole career in themselves. There are those who wear them during the day, but they don't wear a whole strip; they just wear smaller sections. You have to place them carefully using *dark-toned Duo adhesive.* But don't plan on wearing them until you've practiced a couple of times. If you want to dazzle 'em by playing up the eyes as your best feature, you should attach these small pieces of lash over your eyeliner. If you get the pieces of lash really close to the eyeliner, people won't know you have them on. They add a lot of allure. Another sneaky way to wear lashes is to apply them only to the outer corners of your upper lash.

Whichever way you decide to wear them, here's the drill. First, you need to buy the right ones. The most natural-looking ones, which are good to start with, are #747, carried by most beauty supply outlets. They come in short, medium, and long. Be sure to get the *upper lash* because there are lower lashes as well. I like MAC's Raquel Lashes or Maybelline Wisp; both are irregular, with short and long mixed together, and aren't evenly placed on the base like a picket fence. Just finding the right pair is half the battle. Browns will probably look good if you're blonde. Dark brown or black will suit brunettes.

False eyelashes are often too long and need some trimming. I do it with cuticle scissors. Some beauty supply stores have qualified staff who will help you with this. I usually trim mine while they are on my eyes, so I can see where they're too long. But some people find that too scary. It takes a steady hand to cut certain hairs without ruining others. Also, the base of the lash is typically too long when you hold it up to your eye. It extends way past the outside corner. So you'll have to cut it yourself. What you need to know is that false eyelashes are tapered, from longer on the outside corners to shorter on the inside near your nose—like the way natural lashes grow. Therefore it's best to cut the longer outside ends and preserve the shorter tapered lashes.

With new lashes, I usually pull off all the sticky stuff from the base that glues them to the box. It's often clumpy and uneven. I line my eyes and put on mascara before applying lashes.

To attach them, squeeze a small amount of Duo adhesive onto a clean surface that is very close at hand. Dip the end of a cuticle stick into the glue and, while holding the lash in one hand, lightly spread the Duo along the base. Put down the stick, and with both hands or a pair of tweezers to help, place the lash as close as possible to the roots of your upper lashes. (Test this placement before applying the glue, to see where it looks best.) Use a clean stick to tap the lash into place.

Once you get your lashes trimmed and trained to the shape of your eye, don't throw them away. You can use them again. Just carefully strip off the dried adhesive and place them back in the box. If at first you don't succeed, try again. You'll get the hang of it.

Lips I always put lip balm on first and then blot off the excess. Before adding color, I make sure that the area next to my lip line is covered with the lighter foundation. Next, using a lip liner, I outline the shape of my mouth to even out the imbalances from one side to the other. In my case, one side is thinner than the other. Inside the liner, I add a flesh-colored lipstick, Bardot from MAC, which I blot with my fingertips. Over that, I add my basic lipstick color from the tube, and this ensures a soft color. Next, I blend the liner with the lip color using a lipstick brush. Then I blot the edges and use a light beige lip liner to soften it. Finally, I powder just the lip line, which softens it further, and apply a frosted lip gloss very sparingly.

A Fashion Face

A fashion look can be great fun for special occasions. It's usually slightly exaggerated in the magazines to get the point across, but it boils down to minor changes which you can incorporate into your regular beauty makeup. Try a change of lip color and the latest gloss, or you can embellish your look with brush-on bronzers and sheen. You can also play up your eye shadow with shimmer and false lashes.

If you're inspired by a magazine photo, let it be a guide to new products and how you might use them. Try adding wing-tipped eyeliner. Experiment with a few ideas before the big night, when there's still time to play. In the final analysis, most trendy tricks are only fun for a one-time event. You can always add bells and whistles for a special occasion, but they're usually too much for everyday wear. Leave the wild exaggerations for rockers like Amy Winehouse and Lady Gaga.

An Everyday Face

You haven't got all day. You're in a rush, running late for an appointment and dreading the traffic. You need to put on your face in record time and get out the door. There are only two keys for doing easy, radiant daytime makeup. The first is to *use the minimum amount you can get away with, for maximum effect.* The second rule is that makeup should always be *perfectly blended,* so it doesn't look painted-by-the-numbers.

Always keep in mind that less is more. In the '60s we used to wear three pairs of eyelashes at a time! It was the style then. But now, when I look back at those photos, I can't believe I had the nerve to do it. The

'60s were a particularly wild time, and we were all influenced by the daring and exuberance of that moment.

If you're a woman under forty-five, you may still get a kick out of the latest trends, but whether you're younger or older, *you should have a basic beauty look that represents you and isn't subject to fashion trends.* This can be achieved with well-cared-for skin and a minimum of makeup. Once you get good at doing *your* face, you can change it by incorporating a nod to fashion so that your look doesn't get dated or left behind. Just don't abandon your basic face, which is the best foundation to build on.

Your Face in Under Twenty Minutes

After washing and applying toning lotion, moisturize and add some lip balm. If you use whitening strips, apply them directly after brushing your teeth, so that by the time you're finished with your makeup, your teeth will be a little brighter.

Before you do your eyes, use a Q-tip to clear away any moisture under your lower lashes and above the upper lash line. Add a touch of powder to those areas. This will keep you from smudging your eyeliner. Apply a pencil liner close to the lower lash and above the upper lashes at the outside corners. Blend with a Q-tip. Or, if you prefer, instead of a liner, brush on a touch of eye shadow next to the lower lash so the eyes don't look naked. (If you possess luscious lashes you may not need liner every day.) Just curl your lashes and dust lightly with powder. Apply mascara. Use a lash brush to remove any clumps. Liquid liner on the upper lid is optional; make sure to soften it with a Q-tip.

Put on your foundation with a sponge as usual. For an even quicker application, just cover the darkness under the eyes, around the mouth, and your trouble spots with a light, neutral foundation or concealer.

Your quick eyebrow shaping will depend on your brows. If you have sparser brows, use light strokes with a sharpened eyebrow pencil, only where they're thin or uneven. Or try a wedged brow brush and apply cake brow filler. You can also use a combination of both. Brush lightly over your handiwork with a brow brush to soften.

If you have lovely thick eyebrows, be sure they are well plucked and groomed. This is best done the night before, but you do have time for strays. For a fuller brow, you may want to use an eyebrow gel on a brow comb, which will gently separate the hairs and add a slight sheen. It's a matter of taste and time.

For superquick lips, apply a tinted lip balm and blot. Or, to achieve fuller lips, use a natural-colored liner to outline your mouth. Blot off the excess liner. Then fill in with a flesh-color lipstick as a light base before you apply your regular color. The base softens the tone of whatever lipstick you use. Blend the liner and lipstick together. The lip liner shouldn't be evident. Now do a light dusting of translucent powder along the very edge of the mouth, so your liner doesn't run. Finish off with gloss, if you like. (Try using gloss in the center of the bottom lip only.) Lastly, whisk on a fresh colored blusher. Put a dab of foundation on your foundation sponge and blend. *Et voilà!* You're ready to face the day.

If you have time for one last thing, quickly sponge on a warmer-toned foundation. This is for color, not coverage. Just whisk it on over the forehead, the lower cheek, and under the chin. It is slimming to the face and makes you look lightly tanned.

You'll like the finished results. Wearing a little makeup is uplifting to those around you, too. It's like wearing a smile.

Mirror, Mirror

Day after day we see the same face in the mirror, and sometimes we need a little inspiration to get things rolling. It helps to think of making up as an expression of who you are. It should reflect how you feel about yourself. I'm convinced that beauty and style demonstrate an attitude toward life and what role you see yourself playing in it.

Before I developed my look, I went through a period when I hadn't found myself. I was thrown into the spotlight overnight and suddenly invited to attend a string of sophisticated affairs that were overwhelming for an unseasoned girl from a beach community. I was racked with uncertainty about how the world would perceive me. When in doubt, I had to fake it.

There were those people who influenced me, but very few sparked my imagination. I was hungry for some expert direction when I met the formidable Diana Vreeland, the legendary doyenne of *Vogue* magazine and probably its most celebrated editor in chief. She was also someone I greatly admired. Take it from me, in the history of beauty and fashion, she was a phenomenon!

I had just appeared on the cover of *Vogue* magazine when I was exposed to Her Highness in person for the first time. My knees were shaking as I found myself sitting across from Diana's lofty presence. We were surrounded by the blood-red lacquered walls of her office in Manhattan. It was like being in a decadent jewel box. She looked like Nefertiti, with her black hair slicked back into an enormous beehive. I felt extraordinarily plain, but she was kind. She complimented me on the photo spread Richard Avedon had just shot and on my meteoric rise to stardom, all the while sizing me up with her ancient-elephant eyes. Sensing that I felt rather fragile beneath her gaze, she offered this unforgettable observation about herself and her view of beauty: "There are millions of pretty girls and models. But beauty is an attitude! I am not, of course, a conventional beauty. And yet, when I look at my reflection in the mirror each morning, I see an empress, and that's what I become." Wow! She left me breathless. I never forgot what she said.

What she was getting at is that *we are who we think we are*. I will always love her for that, and for her completely uninhibited bravado. She was queen of the grand gesture, and the inspiration behind the massive photographic spreads that appeared in *Vogue* during an epic era that changed the face of fashion. She made millions of women look beyond the makeup and clothes and dream. She never saw just what *was*. She always saw *endless possibilities*.

Every woman should be that way. When she looks into a mirror before she starts to make herself up, she should allow herself to dream a little and realize her possibilities. Let's face it . . . *it's who you are under all that makeup that makes the difference.* Otherwise, it's like a paint job on a car. It might look great, but has nothing to do with what's under the hood.

ELEVEN

Personal Style

CALL IT FLAIR, PANACHE, CHIC — STYLE IS THAT indefinable quality that sets one apart from the herd. And like a fingerprint, it's unique, individual, and can't be faked.

There are no rules or specific steps to achieve a sense of style. Indeed, style is usually the result of someone breaking the rules of convention, not randomly, but as a means of self-expression. Basically, it originates in doing what comes naturally. Or, as Quentin Crisp once put it, "Style is being yourself, but on purpose."

Who Are You?

Now, that can be a tricky question. Not only is it important to know exactly who you are, you also need the confidence to show it. Having style means going out on a limb and revealing something personal when most people are shying away from expressing themselves too freely. They opt for playing it safe and are afraid of letting secrets out of the closet. Having style takes a fair degree of confidence and an extra pinch of chutzpah! Granted, you may want to edit your personality a bit for public consumption, but do it without censoring *all* the idiosyncrasies that make you different from everybody else.

I'll never forget some priceless words of advice from the great Italian director Vittorio De Sica, who directed Sophia Loren in many of her Italian comedies. In the '60s, early in my film career, we were working together in Rome, and I was still groping for my own sense of style both on camera and in my personal life. I felt that the press was scrutinizing my every move as a newcomer, and I'd become painfully self-conscious. I wanted to talk right, walk right, say my lines perfectly, look flawless, and somehow mask the fact that I was still very green and inexperienced. It seemed impossible to live up to public expectations. It was tying me in knots!

Although eager to please on the set, I was given very little direction as an actress and was losing confidence when *il Commandatore* (the Commander, which was how everyone referred to Vittorio) came to my rescue. He took me aside one day, smiled kindly, and said, "My darling girl, why are you trying to change yourself?" I stammered something about needing to be perfect because everyone was watching me. He threw his head back and laughed. "Ahhh, I see," he said sweetly in his simpatico Italian accent. "Please, my darling, do not try to be perfect — *because the defect is very important.*" I was so relieved. It was the best thing he could have said to me. He opened my eyes to the fact that my authentic self, with all its flaws, real or imagined, was the most important quality I had to offer.

Less Than Perfect

As I was settling down to write this chapter on *personal style*, I have to confess that I truly didn't feel up to the task. I usually check out the magazines and websites of my favorite designers to see what's happening, as well as the windows and racks at fine stores to shop for new ideas. But I haven't been interested lately, because none of it matters if my zippers won't go up! After all, I can't be stylish when I'm too zaftig, which is a nice way of saying too fat. But I have excuses! First, my neck went out while writing this book, because I was somehow sitting in the wrong position, even in my state-of-the-art ergonomic chair. Then I tore my rotator cuff and fell and broke my toe . . . twice!

Right now, because of sitting day after day at this *bleeping* computer over a period of nine months—like giving birth—I've put on fifteen extra "writing pounds." On days when I can't fit into any of my clothes, I ask myself if this project is really worth it. I've written every word myself . . . no ghostwriter! Ugh. It's like heart surgery through the feet! I have the greatest respect for professional writers. They deserve a purple heart. Writing is a bitch, and deadlines can make you ugly.

In the meantime, I am forced to deal with how nothing in my closet fits. If you think I walk around perfect *all* the time, think again.

How to Hide the Bulge

If you're interested, and by chance find yourself in a similar predicament, I'll tell you how I manage when I'm not my ideal weight. First of all, *I have three different sets of clothes in my closet.* Doesn't everybody? I have slim, medium, and *OMG!* If the last size starts to fit snugly, I'm in trouble. Big trouble. Here are my guidelines:

✓ *I don't wear tight jeans—especially in white— unless I have an over-blouse or top that covers the hips.*

✓ *I wear my beautiful Versace slacks, which I've had for five years and which never go out of style. They're a classic cut that flows when I walk. They go with everything and always look good.*

✓ *I wear long-sleeve, usually cotton-jersey tops that don't fit skintight, but aren't baggy either. I recommend wearing short-sleeve tops for comfort under a jacket. The tops I choose are V-neck or scoop neck. This keeps the focus higher on* the body. People look at your face and chest area first, not at the middle or trunk of your body. A crew neck makes your head look small and your body bigger. If, however, you have petite proportions and are not busty, you can probably get away with it. Regardless of what top I choose, in the majority of cases I like to wear a jacket—unless it's a scorcher. It adds an upscale flair. I have a favorite YSL jacket that I've had for ten years, which I bought for nicer occasions. But now I wear it casually during the day with jeans. It always rocks.

✓ For casual dressing in warm weather, I turn to jean jackets in blue, stonewash, or tan. I wear these with my slacks to dial things down for more casual occasions. Or I wear a lightweight leather jacket, or even my motorcycle jacket for cool evenings. In summer, I like to wear Theory's white cotton, two-button blazer, with a colorful camisole top or striped shell. (I save the matching white cotton pants for periods when I'm slim.) I add sandals and a summer tote, in patent, straw, or canvas, or a fun clutch. As I said, I stay away from white pants when my weight is iffy, because they just highlight every bulge. Instead I pair the white jacket with darker pants, or even with my black stretch Ralph Lauren jeans.

✓ Seersucker jackets also look good during summer, if you add a simple top and a nice easy-fit pair of pants. I used to have a seersucker suit for summer by Norma Kamali that eventually got ruined. I always keep one eye open for another. My basic jackets usually fit me at any weight. It's the pants that vary.

✓ When it comes to weight problems, squeezing into a favorite dress may be too dodgy. Perhaps you can wear an empire-style dress, with the seam under the bust and an A-line skirt. It's more forgiving. When in doubt, pass on it. Remember, a dress always gets more attention . . . even when you don't want it. When it's too tight, you're never comfortable. I myself wait until my hourglass figure reappears. Stick to separates in the meantime.

At Normal Weight

At normal weight, here are some good staples.

✓ If you've got good legs, a skirt, top, and jacket can work with pumps or sexy sandals. Learn how to cross your legs so that your skirt is not halfway up your thighs. Longer skirts can work too, if you prefer.

✓ There are several options for the winter. Latex leggings, which are in right now, can be worn with a long sweater and fabulous boots. If you're trim enough, try a minidress with leggings. If that's too much for you, choose a longer skirt with a long slit in the back or side. Wear flesh or smokey-colored hose or fishnets, if you dare, and your favorite boots. If you wear a longish sweater as a top over pants, tights, or a skirt, consider a designer belt, slung low on the hip, which usually makes you look taller and slimmer. It's your call.

✓ Another idea is a longer vest worn over an untucked blouse, or over a long-sleeve jersey, several inches longer than the vest. Whether this works or not depends on the proportion of the vest.

✓ A poncho can be fun over pants and a long-sleeve top.

✓ Try wearing a smoothing garment under thin sweaters so bra lines or bulges are not visible. These are available at most department stores in the foundations department.

Never Enough Shoes

Your shoes and handbags need not be an exact match, but should coordinate with and enhance your wardrobe. For formal affairs, this means a pair of dressy heels, which can be classic pumps, open-toed or sandals. They don't have to be miles high if you're tall. But three inches or more for a long gown really adds to the effect. With a cocktail dress they are also a must, if your feet can stand it. They make tanned legs look great. You can wear toeless hose if you need the coverage and support.

You should also own a pair of boots. They can be knee or ankle length, worn under your pants or with a skirt. And you'll want some daytime sandals, wedgies, and/or espadrilles. For casual wear in warm weather, you can also get away with a metallic sandal.

Every woman needs comfortable flats to wear every day to knock around in. You should also have some cross-trainers that you wear for exercise. My sneakers often double as mall shopping and errand shoes. They really save my feet. You can pair them with cargo pants, jeans, or any easy, knock-around pants, like those from the Da Nang clothing line, which I wear with flip-flops on vacation in the Caribbean. But any casual, roomier pants will work with flat shoes or sandals. To be comfortable or to be beautiful, that is the question. The goal is to be both.

The length of your trousers can be an issue when it comes to footwear. I have longer pants to wear with higher heels and boots. I also have shorter, more casual pants to wear with flats, because otherwise the hem will drag along the floor.

High Heels

I happen to be one of those women who has a shoe fetish. I love them and have more than I can wear. Sometimes I am forced to take a pass on the really death-defyingly steep ones—if they already hurt in the store, I don't walk out in them. Gorgeous as high heels can be, they pitch my balance too far forward and occasionally throw my lower back and hip out. So no, I can't always wear them.

When I was younger, I even danced onstage in five-inch heels. I was ready to suffer for beauty, but there comes a point when the accumulated suffering of a lifetime reaches a dead end. I still have some killer shoes, but I only wear them when I can calculate exactly how long I'll be standing on a hard surface before I can reach carpet. Cement and marble are the worst, so I don't put on my stilettos until the last minute before I get in the car. On the red carpet, I usually wear platform heels under long gowns. I find them more comfortable, and I don't have to sacrifice height. And yet, by the end of the evening my feet are burning. A life of glamour is devoted to enduring discomfort. Ask any model. The big bucks are for the pain and suffering . . . and the starving.

These days, shoes that make the most potent fashion statement are usually platform heels and dominatrix-style gladiator straps, reminiscent of an Amazonian vixen. They're smokin', and I like them for dress-up. But it's worrisome to think that with my strong shoulders and prominent cheekbones I might be in danger of being cast in a role outside my comfort zone. I don't like being seen as predatory. I'm looking for a dance partner, not a slave. Although I do have a pair in my closet if the spirit moves me, I haven't found the right moment to wear them yet. They'd be perfect for Adam Lambert when he tours with Queen. But when I look back at the time when I danced in five-inch heels in Vegas and Atlantic City and did fourteen shows a week, all I can say is, What was I thinking?

Protecting Your Feet

Extreme footwear puts added stress on our feet, so I take steps to protect them and preserve my posture by wearing orthotic insoles in my shoes. I need them to support my ankles and high arches. I have a pair of custom-made orthotics that I've worn in my sneakers for workouts and walking since the '80s. They even make them for high heels, but I never seem to wear mine. Living in New York, when my back kept going out as I walked through the city, my chiropractor recommended I see a podiatrist. It seems that a large percentage of former dancers have this problem. At the chiro's office, I always run into dancers I know from Broadway.

At the podiatrist's, it was pointed out that when I stand straight in bare feet, my arches pronate and my feet roll slightly inward toward each other. This throws my alignment off and can cause back, hip, and neck problems, especially if you are an active person. It's like the domino effect, moving up the body from feet to neck. An orthotic device can support your arch and also equalize your leg length. All in all, it keeps the feet aligned, so that your ankles, knees, and hips can stay in balance.

The wear and tear from dancing, workouts, and even yoga and just staying active is a factor that has to be addressed sooner or later. Dancers and athletes usually know how to treat these conditions so they can extend the longevity of their professional careers. But from your mid-forties on, it's important to be aware of ways to correct your spine alignment, which protects the quality of life. When I started to have trouble, the adjustment to my feet and, subsequently, my posture, changed my life. So even if you're younger, don't let it go.

The most important thing I have to tell you is: Save those feet. They deserve respect. If you cannot wear higher shoes, don't injure yourself for beauty's sake. You should adjust the length of your skirts and pants accordingly. If you have problems walking or back problems, you might want to examine the way you balance your weight on your feet. There may be something that can be done to help. If the remedy is prescribed by a licensed doctor, it will probably be covered by insurance. Take care of your body, and it will take care of you.

Handbags and Purses

During 2009, the huge handbag craze, with matching price tags, finally peaked. Every woman I know has enough of those bags to last a decade.

I still like the ones I have and will probably get good use out of them, but the market was awfully saturated. It was a period when I felt like there wasn't any radical new direction in fashion, so accessories took center stage. A wardrobe of status purses, belts of all sizes, and spectacular shoes made all the difference. They were must-haves to achieve *the look*. It was a time of extravagance, when there was an underlying premonition that such excess couldn't last forever. I think a return to less-extreme handbags, to go with a more streamlined silhouette, is what's happening now. At least that's the direction I'm headed in. The '60s retro styles are still a factor for teens and the younger crowd, but dressing like an adult has actually become stylish these days.

Where once there were limited choices of purses for different occasions, now there is an endless assortment of them. Fortunately, plenty of fashionable bags can be had for reasonable prices. I wish designers would strike a happy medium between too much room, which means that you can't find anything, and not enough room, which means you never have what you need. We'll probably achieve world peace sooner.

Fashion Trends

Fashion is meant to influence and inspire, but don't let it bully you. You don't have to go along for the ride and become a "fashion victim." After all, in the end it's your choice; you're the buyer. In the final analysis, *you're* the one who dictates what's *in* and what's *out* by exercising your prerogative — not the other way around

Are you on a tight budget? Not to worry. You don't need a lot of money to dress well or have great style and class. In fact, more fashion sins are committed against good taste by the *nouveaux riches* than by those who have to make choices based on budget limitations and practical need. Remember, *style depends on a unique idea of how to put different elements together*. The proof is often in the personal details. You can't buy a creative sense. Great style is like common currency and works at any time and any place. It breaks through social and economic barriers like a hot knife through butter. Anyone can play.

Quite often, fashion designers take their inspiration from different cultural traditions. They create whole collections based on the way everyday people dress in, say, Russia, China, Africa, Paris in the '20s, Bali, Indonesia, India, Tibet, or Spain. Their sources of inspiration are endless. It's refreshing to note that some of the world's top designers are heavily influenced by the rural customs of peasants or fishermen from various countries. They study how they layer their clothing, tie their scarves, and drape their bodies with fabrics. They take note of what combinations of colors, fabrics, and accessories these unjaded ethnic cultures use. Take a cue from this. Never feel that you need to be unduly "sophisticated" to be stylish.

I'm not suggesting that you wear a folk-dancing costume to your job interview, but there's always something in everyone's background, travel experiences, or exposure to different periods and cultures that can feed your imagination. This could be the key to your personal style. So take the time to soak up all the ideas around you.

Developing Your Style

What do you *want* to look like—and what, realistically, *can* you pull off? Reality is the great equalizer. You may aspire to look like your favorite actress, model, or someone else you admire. Embrace that influence, but *don't play copycat*. It gets in the way of exploring who you really are.

At the same time, you must give full rein to your more adventurous side. There's no need to suppress your impulses at the first sign of doubt. Your inspiration might be sparked by a magazine photo or just an idea in your head. Either way it can be useful when you want to try something new. It's fun to experiment! A girl also needs to see what doesn't work. It's every bit as important as knowing what does. Trying different things arms you with valuable information.

While you're in the process of pulling together a new look, it's great to get advice from a friend. After all, we do care what others think. So, if you're feeling in need of an objective point of view, there's no harm in asking for one, from someone reliable. Listen and weigh what is said, before making your purchases.

Creative play for all grown-ups is essential. It's particularly stimulating for anyone who is developing an individual style. Go to the theater, read a good novel, pore over art books, listen to all kinds of music, wander through flea markets, thumb through history books, travel, and visit museums. Above all, allow yourself to daydream. These are not trivial pastimes. They are a means of making connections, of gathering inspiration and energy. You can't invent anything of consequence— much less reinvent yourself—without exposing yourself to life.

Colorful Connections

Your use of color obviously has a lot to do with your style. Some people seem to shy away from bright or dramatic color and are always a vision in beige. That can be a style statement too, but I've always been attracted to vivid color. Fortunately, with my olive skin, I can get away with wearing a variety of different tones. I like oranges and coral, hot pinks, turquoise, and sky blue, certain reds without too much blue in them, and lavender. But my favorite colors are black and white. I love the graphic pop of either one. Oddly enough, technically they are both considered *noncolors*. White, which is the presence of all colors of light, and black, which is the total absence of light, are at opposite extremes of the spectrum. This is a fact that I learned in a context I'm not likely to forget.

When I was shooting *Myra Breckenridge,* in 1968, I had a scene with Mae West, the Queen of Hollywood in the black-and-white era. Mae was famous for her risqué dialogue and was also known for wearing white. The costume designer Theodora Van Runkle confirmed that Ms. West would be wearing a custom-made white creation, designed by the fabulous Edith Head, for our much anticipated scene together. Mae would be swathed in alabaster white, with one slash of black streaming down from her sizable hat. Van Runkle, who designed my clothes for the film, had already become famous for creating Faye Dunaway's chic '30s look in *Bonnie and Clyde* and was everyone's darling. She was dripping with talent.

For our upcoming "clash of the titans," Theodora designed a sophisticated black velvet gown for me, with a slim, full-length skirt that skimmed the body all the way to the floor. A matching long-sleeved bolero jacket fit very snugly at the top and boasted an explosion of white ruffles at the neck and the cuff of each sleeve. She was inspired by a vintage photo of Garbo, no less, and the whole effect was elegance itself, topped off by a black velvet hat with a thin whisper of a veil and a sprig of dramatic cock feathers as a finishing touch. *C'était très soigné.* The look was absolutely on target for Myra, as she was always emulating stars of an earlier epoch.

When the day of the scene arrived, this exquisite costume disappeared from my dressing room. I had just put on black hose and a garter belt, since Theodora suggested that I have period underwear for the role; and I was standing there in these undergarments and my shoes and hat, fully made up and ready for my dress. Ruth, my dresser, opened the wardrobe closet and went pale.

"Where's the dress? It's not here!" She was absolutely certain that she'd hung it in my dressing room first thing in the morning; and now it was gone!

As it turned out, Mae had gotten wind that I was wearing a black dress and gone bananas. She demanded that the producer confiscate this gown from my dressing room. Scared to death that she might walk off, he had obliged. Apparently, Mae had it written into her contract that no actress in the movie who appeared on camera with her could wear a *noncolor*. That was *her* exclusive domain. The gown finally reappeared seven hours later, following a little standoff on my end. And it was eventually decided that I could not appear in the same frame of film as Madam. In other words, there would never be a shot of the two of us together. Now you understand why I can never forget the distinction between colors and *noncolors*, imposed on me by Ms. West.

It was much ado about nothing, as far as I was concerned; and I didn't like being bullied. Still, I felt sympathetic to the aging legend, who was seventy-seven at the time and had never made a Technicolor movie. I arrived on set to shoot our scene with two dozen roses for Mae, as a peace offering. She stared at me blankly and said, "Thanks, kid. Uh . . . What did ya say your name was?"

Long after *Myra* wrapped, I learned that every color has a significant meaning, and that is why we are attracted to them. They speak to us in a subliminal way and say something about our individual spiritual nature. I'm sure that you've noticed the effect that certain colors have on you, but perhaps, like me, you'd like to know what they mean.

Red: passion, fiery emotion, and, of course, sex and matters of the heart.

Blue: the color of communication, truth, and honesty.

Purple and *dark blue*: the colors of royalty.

Green: the color of healing and cleansing. It reminds me of algae and chlorophyll. That's probably why I don't like to wear it very often. In fact, I'm not at all attracted to darker greens. But give me a lovely, vibrant emerald green, and I'm happy to be healed and cleansed.

Black: the color of mystery, intrigue, and spirits of the night.

White: purity and power.

Lavender, lilac, and *mauve tones*: the colors of spirituality and imagination.

Yellow: the color of youth, newness, and rebirth.

It's undeniable that color has a lot of emotion attached to it. It has the power to create an atmosphere and mood. Your choice of color can calm you, excite you, bolster your confidence, and give you an unforgettable entrance. If you are comfortable wearing color, it can often lift the morale of the people around you. Whether you go monotone, pastel, or vivid, if used to maximum effect, the color of your clothes is bound to leave a lasting impression.

Dress to Impress

Everyone is eager to make a good impression. Dressing well can be an asset. It can help you win friends and influence people. It may also help you get that job, land a promotion, or win hearts. But how you dress should also lift your spirits as part of the bargain. It should bring out your personality, not eclipse you. Don't let the clothes wear you.

Whether you're stylin' for a professional occasion, a social engagement, or a hot date, clothes should be an expression of who you are. And yet, good manners and the right clothes only take you so far. The takeaway that makes you memorable is your personality and attitude. That's what people are left with after you are gone. It's the overall effect that puts you in their mind and makes you unforgettable.

It's time to reinforce your confidence and "express yourself," to repeat Madonna's mantra. Your personal style can improve your reputation or uphold the good one you already have. Although you need to look good, you should also be comfortable and at ease when relating to other people and participating in the activity you came for. Allow yourself to dress with a sense of humor by injecting an element of whimsy into the mix.

Your accessories can play a part in this. Just the way you tie a scarf or wear a signature necklace, rings, bracelets, watch, and earrings is always an opportunity to say something about your attitude or your eye for the unusual.

I happen to have a thing for men's hats. I collect them like shoes. I have a straw fedora for summer and a felt one for fall. I also collect berets, and French cheese-cutter caps. I love all kinds of cowboy hats for any season. Some girls look cute in large-brimmed, floppy hats with jeans or a summer skirt. They have these hats in felt, too, for the fall. For me, a hat serves many purposes. It shades me from UV rays, covers up bad hair days, adds allure, and looks unique. Hats are just one way of saying something personal about yourself—and they're great for travel when your hair goes limp on the plane.

Shop 'Til You Drop

Stylish women put a fair amount of time and effort into preparing a wardrobe of essentials that will carry them through their social, personal, and professional lives. I sympathize with those of you who have limited time, because that's the boat I'm usually in. But without preparation you will always be caught off guard without the appropriate thing to wear.

You need to assemble a practical, basic wardrobe that works in a variety of different situations; and there's no reason in the world to believe that you have to start from scratch. You no doubt have some pieces in your wardrobe *right now* that are already working for you. By rethinking these tried-and-true staples, you can give yourself a fresh new look. Whether or not you've already taken care of getting into shape, there will be some clothes that make you feel great and others that don't. Stick to the ones that flatter you.

It's assumed that if you're female, you were born to shop. For many, that's true. But others, like me, resent spending a lot of valuable time trying on clothes when they could be doing something else. It can become an exhausting ritual and frustrating process. Whether you're young or old, shopping can be quite daunting unless you have something specific in mind. When I shop, I break it down into four steps, so that I don't get overwhelmed.

1. Research. Take a look around. Go window shopping and look everywhere, from high-end department stores to discount fashion places, so you know what's out there. Check out your favorite designers at stores or on the Internet and take note of the prices. A $3,000 designer handbag may have a look-alike for a fraction of the cost. Style is not about money; it's about choices. It's your chance to prove that you're a clever girl with a signature look that seems very natural and uncontrived.

2. Organize. It's a good idea to arrange the clothes in your closet according to category and by color within each group. This will enable you to look through your wardrobe and see what you have that you still like and that is still in style. Put those items together in one section of your closet. Put warm-weather clothes in one section and cold-weather apparel in another. I have a section for dressy clothes and one for separates. I keep all my jackets together and all pants together. I do the same thing with suits, shirts, blouses, and tops; but I have a separate section just for camisoles, organized by color.

3. Itemize. Decide what items in your closet you need to augment *before* you begin to shop. You may need to recheck after you've seen what's out there. Target the stores that have the items you're looking for. This narrows it down quite a bit.

4. Self-appraisal. There are practical questions you need to ask yourself before you begin shopping for clothes that look great on your body type.

- ✓ How tall are you? Are you tall and slim or tall and full-bodied?
- ✓ Do you have a big bust or a small bust?
- ✓ Do you have wide hips or narrow hips?
- ✓ What do you look like walking away? Do you need to hide your "caboose" or show it off to best advantage?
- ✓ Are you pear-shaped, meaning narrow across the shoulders or across the bust and larger below?
- ✓ Are you short or long-waisted? Do you have a defined waistline or are you less curvy?
- ✓ What is your coloring? Do you have an ivory, olive, café au lait, or mocha complexion? Whether you have light or dark skin, what exact color tone is your face? Some darker skin is more yellow or brown, more grayish or possesses reddish overtones. Learn to choose the most attractive colors for your skin tone. Many natural blondes stick to neutral shades, because intense saturated colors are too strong for their paler complexion (unless they have a tan, of course).

✓ What is your hair color—blonde, brunette, auburn, or redhead?

✓ What is the color of your eyes, and do you want to play them up?

✓ Do you need to cover your arms or do you want to feature a set of buffed biceps?

✓ What is the shape of your legs? What's a good length for you?

Practical knowledge of what you have to work with saves a lot of time. Know your limitations, because we all have them. This helps you to focus on what you are looking for. Shopping can be very confusing and tiring. Personally, it's not my favorite way to spend an afternoon, until I start to find something that works. It always takes some persistence.

Figure Flaws and Foundations

Because of the growing boomer demographic, various types of foundation garments to cope with every need have become available in recent years. Don't feel self-conscious about visiting these departments. Even actresses in their twenties are wearing Spanx or similar control garments. Here's a list of options to choose from:

Push-up bras — to enhance your cleavage.

Minimizer bras — to downplay a large bosom.

High-waisted Spanx — to smooth your body under clothes, from under the breast to midthigh.

Body suits — to smooth your entire torso from under the arms to midthigh.

Under-bust corsets — These are boned cinchers, which fit over the shoulders with armholes. They fasten with hooks down the front, under your bust, allowing the bust to protrude above.

The boned corset cinches in the entire torso, including the sides of the breasts, sculpting the waist and holding in the top of the hip above the buttocks.

Waist cinchers — These attach just around the middle of the torso and have boning to minimize the size of the waist.

Hip and leg Spanx — for smoothing the body under a pair of pants.

Spanx are thinner and harder to detect under formfitting clothes than the old-fashioned girdles of an earlier decade. If a foundation garment includes bones and hooks and eyes, it may be visible under close-fitting dresses or stretch fabrics. To camouflage a heavy-duty foundation, try wearing a Spanx smoother over it. However, if comfort is an issue and you are going out to eat, it's not worth it. Find a different outfit.

Cut and Fit Are Everything!

Always pay close attention to those designers and brands that cut clothes for your particular body type. The only way to know is to try them on. They don't have to be expensive fashion houses, but the cut has to work on your body. Shopping by a designer line that is right for you is half the battle. Once I find a designer that works for me, I go back to that line of clothes again and again like a homing pigeon. It's akin to having a stylist on call, because they usually have other items that will coordinate nicely with what you buy. If you can't afford everything all at once, get the most important piece or pieces and come back for the extra items later. Stores will usually order your size if it's not in stock.

When deciding what to buy, I find it's better to invest in a few high-quality well-made pieces that fit beautifully. One basic cornerstone is a sharp jacket that can be worn with a top, blouse, or shirt. Choose one that will coordinate beautifully with the pants and skirts that are already in your wardrobe. Or get a great-fitting suit. Now you have the nucleus of a new look you can build on.

If you can't rely on a particular designer, a good boutique whose buyer knows your taste is indispensable. Most department stores now arrange things in boutique sections so you can see what goes with what. When you have to put together a whole outfit by running from one department to the next, it's the pits.

My Looks and Limits

I myself have several favorite designers: some for classic staples, which are the most important, others for more avant-garde and sexy looks, and others who do beautiful evening wear and party dresses. But I always keep my eye on the field, for that exceptional find. There are so many great designers that occasionally, I play hooky and shop somewhere else, but I count on my regulars. Among them are: Michael Kors, Dolce & Gabbana, Ralph Lauren, Donna Karan, Armani, Versace, Escada, and Oscar de la Renta. In addition to their couture lines, they all have ready-to-wear collections with accessible prices.

With the popularity of *Project Runway*, the public is privy to the creative process behind inventing a season of beautiful new styles. And yet, when a designer discontinues my favorite cuts in favor of a new trend, it breaks my heart. I'm usually loyal to my favorite fashion houses and give them the first chance to fit me each time around. But for practical reasons, it's best to have some backup.

I don't begrudge designers their innovations, but I so wish every line had a few core basics in new fabrics with fresh detailing that loyal followers could rely upon. New styles are fun, but so often the latest look is kind of weird; for example, gathered hemlines and puffy balloon skirts. This stuff is more for *fashionistas*. It isn't designed to make most women look their best.

When I choose clothes, I'm very aware that a good fit is essential. Like many women over fifty, I often have a hard time finding something attractive to wear. Not everything I try on fits like a glove. There's a lot to consider with my body, so I'm not inclined toward overtly sexy looks. I prefer the contrast of tailored clothes on a voluptuous figure.

I have broad shoulders, and what has affectionately been called "a crowd in the balcony," so I need a jacket that allows for my frontage. I also like the jacket to have room in the shoulders, allowing the arm gusset to settle into place without any stress pulls. I look best in single-breasted jackets with narrow-cut waists. If you have an hourglass figure, this kind of jacket might suit you as well. If the shoulder doesn't fit or the bosom looks over-stuffed, it's a wash.

Unfortunately, I don't look good in short, boxy jackets. They don't flatter my curves. However, if you're one of those lucky women who are smaller busted, those short, boxy jackets will probably look chic and great on you. Think Jackie O or Audrey Hepburn or, lately, Victoria Beckham and Katie Holmes. Some women who are narrow across the back but still have breasts can also pull off this look.

Three Essential Pieces

When you think about it, separates are as simple as one, two, three. Here's an easy formula that might help you organize your shopping needs in an uncomplicated way. Once you know you need the basic three items—a *pair of pants, a top, and a jacket*—your brain doesn't have to work so hard. Ditto with a skirt look. There are just three basic pieces: *skirt, top, and jacket*. You can't miss. Simply substitute the pieces with variations on the theme. For example, wear trousers instead of jeans. Or substitute a T-shirt for the blouse, or wear a low-cut, close-fitting top that works comfortably under your jacket. For the younger set, a bustier under a tailored jacket or short blazer might work well for a hot date. By the way, you don't need to fasten your jacket closed. It usually looks better open. The garment should settle easily over your torso. If your jacket is too tight, the front will swing open like a couple of barn doors.

Other options are a lightweight sweater or shrug instead of a jacket, for warm weather. Or bring a shawl to drape around your shoulders. Restaurants and theaters have air-conditioning that can cause a chill. You might also consider something in leather, based on an aviator, hunting, or motorcycle jacket. You can pair either of these with pants or a skirt. Women who are more full-figured might try wearing a longer skirt and a softer, unstructured jacket or sweater.

Covering Your Neck

If you're like Nora Ephron and hate your neck, try draping a soft scarf around your throat. Learn to tie it artfully, with flair, not like a tourniquet. I have a good neck, knock on wood, but I still like scarves. I used to take a Liberty scarf and fold it over until it was two inches wide. Then I'd twist it and wrap it around my neck, tie it in a square knot and tuck the ends under on either side. You could do the same with a silk scarf, or tie it in a cravat. You could also merely turn your collar up, like the late, great, Kate Hepburn. One actress I know always wears something at the neck. She has necklaces altered to fit like chokers so that her neck is camouflaged by the use of a charming accessory. It has become a trademark of her style.

Whatever the case, don't be afraid to experiment with your jewelry choices and with draping and tying scarves. Many department stores have sales people who are good at helping and can at least start you off. Or get a copy of *Elle* magazine. Because the French do accessories extremely well. Whatever you wear around your neck should look natural and not tortured.

The Little Black Dress and Others

When it comes to black dresses, I usually buy a sheath style with a matching short jacket or shrug, if possible. For me, this style of dress should have a stretch fit, whether it's gabardine, wool crepe, or cotton. It makes your figure look even better when you're in top form, and at only slightly less than perfect, you can still wear it. Since the '80s, a large percentage of dresses have been made from amazing stretch fabrics.

The hardest thing to come by is a dynamite black dress, one that works all year round for many occasions. Michael Kors does this kind of dress beautifully. His are flawless and usually have a great fit. And he usually also does them in a range of luscious colors. They are a treasure and reason enough to stay fit.

For evening attire, if you can pull it off, nothing beats a simple dress with a jacket. A well-cut dress in a lovely pastel with a chic hat can take you to a wedding. Sans chapeau, it's perfect for a cocktail party or a dressy dinner, with the right jewelry, shoes, clutch, and delicately beaded wrap.

With few exceptions, I'm not partial to beaded dresses and other flashy numbers. The same goes for other flamboyant outfits. It's true that every so often I stumble upon a gold lamé goddess dress that I have to have. But once you wear something as memorable as that, it is retired from action and goes to the back of the closet. By the time you get back to it, it probably won't fit. I had one such dress custom made for me in Paris by Azzaro. A few years later, when I appeared on Broadway in the musical *Woman of the Year*, I brought it out of retirement. It was perfect. When the curtain went up, a single spotlight hit that gold gown, and it didn't disappoint. I think I weighed 117 pounds at the time.

For most gowns you need to coordinate a wrap. I like to drape a large, dressy shawl around and over one shoulder. This works well for evening if you don't have a fabulous Donna Karan evening coat.

How to Be Elegantly Sexy

If you're single and are trying to increase your chances of connecting with the right man, you might get a case of butterflies just thinking about what you'll wear to meet him. But that's not uncommon and will pass as soon as you start shopping! Women are used to shopping to impress other women, so it's nerve-racking when the focus turns toward dressing to please that special man. The best way to deal with doubt is to put your energy into getting back into the swing of things!

Remember, there are two kinds of people in the world: those who watch from the sidelines and those who play. We all spend time on both sides of that fence, but when the right opportunity presents itself, don't hesitate to make the most of a private romantic encounter. Bring your most seductive side along on every occasion you spend together, and make it special.

Attracting the right man and winning his favor means letting him know that you're a "catch" worthy of his best attentions. What you wear can go a long way to make him aspire to win you. Leave something to the imagination. By all means, be sexy in your choices for the occasion, but not over the top. Too short, too tight, or too low-cut are definitely not advisable; they send the wrong message and smack of too much too soon. Allow him to take the lead and get comfortable with you first. Believe me, he has a very active way of imagining what he cannot see. Men are very stimulated by the visual and get the message loud and clear. So easy does it. You can control the situation by giving the right signals. How you dress says how fast you want things to go. Give yourself a chance to get to know him.

Keep in mind as well that most men like to pursue and win you. Don't rob him of the enjoyment of doing that. When it comes to dressing to go out, it's been my experience that guys prefer to think that the object of their affection is someone exclusive who isn't available to everyone in the room. You're clever enough to strike the right balance between hot and classy, aren't you? Turn up the heat, but don't invite the whole fire department.

In my opinion, Jessica Alba and Heidi Klum usually get it right. Reese Witherspoon *rules* as the nice girl with a ridiculously high IQ and a latent sexy streak. Diane Sawyer is classy, gently probing, intelligent, *and* desirable. Jaclyn Smith is gorgeous and understated; she doesn't need to push it. Diane Keaton is one of a kind, quirky but irresistible.

Some of my personal friends, like the former model Alana Stewart, have an easy elegance and sense of fun that attracts suitors like flies. I'm sure you know women who always seem to pull off every style challenge. Watch and learn. Don't bother letting envy creep in. Instead, take note of how it's done.

Getting the Red Carpet Look

For a red-carpet appearance, lamé, satin crepe, and all the other slinky fabrics are seductive and glamorous. But anything overly shiny catches the light and adds weight on camera. Beading is another story. As an accent, it can be stunning, but overall beading is problematic.

Beading and glitz can add twenty-five pounds to your frame if not done expertly. Bob Mackie is, of course, a genius when it comes to slinky gowns. He knows how to space the beading on the body just right. Otherwise you can look like a house.

Mackie created several spectacular dresses for my Vegas show in the '70s. They were all beaded. He'd fashion them out of flesh-colored soufflé or bias-cut chiffon. The beading was applied strategically to cover the body just enough and catch the light in a flattering way. I looked like I was poured into them. One time he used gold beads in a wheat pattern. This amazing gown was strictly for onstage appearances. Though dazzling under the lights, you could see right through it. I wouldn't dream of wearing it in public.

For another occasion, he placed rows of bugle beads on thin, semi-transparent salmon-colored chiffon, cut on the bias. The secret was leaving a half-inch space between each row of beads. All the beadwork was designed on the bias, too. Talk about glamour! I still have both dresses. In fact, I've saved *all* my costumes, from the doeskin bikini in *One Million Years B.C.* to the wardrobe for my role in *Woman of the Year* on Broadway.

The hitch is, for real life, beading doesn't always work. Who wants to sit on beads all night? Besides, beaded fabric weighs a ton. I think it belongs under the bright lights, not up close and personal, or on my favorite glamazon, Cher. But if you do wear something beaded, select a garment on which the beading is used only as an accent. Also, avoid solid or encrusted sequins and choose bugle beads instead, which are long, flat and more slimming. They were always my preference.

Let's not forget about *le smoking* for a high-voltage appearance. The men's trouser suit was made fashionable for women by Dietrich and later in my generation by the legendary Yves Saint Laurent. It has now become a viable option for black-tie events. An attractive woman can even wear *le smoking* to the Academy Awards. Many of the top designers have created super elegant tuxedos for women's evening attire. I wore a white Tom Ford smoking ensemble with a spectacular Tony Duquette necklace to the *Vanity Fair* Oscars party one year. It looked great and was perfect for me, because I was not inclined to wear a gown. The jacket had a very feminine cut. I wore it over a décolleté top with statement jewelry. It's good to know that you are not obligated to go with a floor-length gown if the spirit doesn't move you. One can find similar smoking ensembles in the better vintage clothing houses and second-hand shops. Many actresses have worn vintage clothes very successfully, even to the Oscars.

Style and the Academy Awards

In my profession, having style of one kind or another is a prerequisite. Sometimes it's even better to be considered kooky and rather tasteless than to have no style at all. As you know, there are a variety of looks adopted by those in the public eye, ranging from the sublime to the ridiculous. Take, for example, the occasion of the annual Academy Awards. Here is an event where personal style — or lack of it — is on display for all it is worth. And here is where approximately 400 million people, the world over, engage in the sport of separating the ones who have it from the ones who don't.

Over the years, I've appeared as a presenter on this televised extravaganza a number of times, with varying degrees of success. The first question asked of every actress who agrees to appear on the Oscar telecast is, "What are you going to wear?" Whether this *should* be top priority is another question. The debate over the awards show as a serious broadcast to honor artistic achievement versus a fashion show *cum* hypefest for the movie industry has yet to be resolved. I think it's safe to say it's both. Obviously, without its star-studded glamour and "style," the Oscars wouldn't be the phenomenon we've come to know and love.

Chances are, even the most faithful movie fan can't remember from year to year who won or lost in the Oscar race, but most viewers recall, down to the last detail, what so-and-so was wearing! Deciding how to dress, then, can be an agonizing dilemma. There's a lot of pressure to get it right. In fact, in the past, some actresses have improved their standing merely with this brief appearance, and some went down for the count. Mistakes in judgment run rampant. Undoubtedly, as far as style is concerned, the Academy Awards show is considered the acid test. But in my day, we didn't have access to stylists, and we paid for Oscar dresses out of our own pocket. Talk about pressure!

These days, for an Oscars telecast, everyone comes off uniformly well groomed and coutured to the max. I myself look forward to seeing colorful personalities, instead of one long monotone of conformity, no matter how tasteful. The fashion police, though they barely seem to qualify for that role, often tend to look quite strange themselves. But they blast away at anyone who wears something too different. I loved it when Barbra Streisand picked up her first Oscar in black see-through bell-bottoms and top. The outfit was sprinkled with glitter and topped off by a white satin Peter Pan collar and cuffs, plus a bow at the neck. That took chutzpah! It was amazing to see. You had to admit, Babs had a great . . . um, derriere!

Years later, Cher, in Bob Mackie's black-feathered, Mohawk headdress and almost-there black-beaded dress, with no sides or back, was fabulosity personified! Bette Midler once made an entrance on the Oscar stage in a full short skirt stiff with crinolines and a strapless bodice. She jiggled her way to the microphone with those trademark itty-bitty steps. As I recall, she said something like, "Good evening everyone. I'm Bette Midler and these . . ." (glancing at her bosoms) "are my girls." Julie Christie wore a miniskirt one year.

I loved Björk for showing up at the Oscars draped in a swan fantasy, feathers and all. Think how banal it would have been had she tried to fit in. Look, I'm not proposing that you drop acid and then get dressed, or force yourself too far out on a limb. But I am in favor of pushing the envelope a little to make a personal statement even if you make some mistakes. I know I did.

In 1970, for my first appearance at the Academy Awards, I chose a rather overblown creation with full sleeves and a Renaissance ballroom skirt in a multicolored tapestry fabric. I should have known better than to venture forth in a gown from a boutique called Granny Takes a Trip! But it was the end of the '60s. I was described by the fashion critic Mr. Blackwell as "a barbecue queen at a bar mitzvah." Not quite the reaction I had hoped for, but it was fun!

In subsequent years, I appeared in considerably less yardage and was received with a more favorable reaction. But on occasion I did raise some eyebrows. One year, Howard Koch, the show's producer, sent word that I was not to wear anything too tight or low-cut. I didn't always obey.

One year I wore a skintight blue-sequined jumpsuit from my Vegas show, because I needed something quick and didn't have enough time to shop. It fit me like a glove and was a proven crowd-pleaser. I flew in on Oscar night, glad that I didn't have to worry about what to wear. The only snag was that when I got into the limo, I discovered that I couldn't sit down in it! How was I to know? I always sang in this outfit standing up! Eventually, I had to unzip it and lie down in the backseat of the limo, all the way to the Dorothy Chandler Pavilion. Never again!

Another year, I wore a draped gown by Norma Kamali that was not tight-fitting but had a plunging neckline. That caused quite a stir. I had to be very careful how I moved. I finally decided the best place for me was the backstage dressing room, where I could relax and wait until needed. I don't recall whether I used two-way tape or not, but my co-presenter, the legendary Kirk Douglas, almost forgot his part of our dialogue that night, he was so distracted. I should have had my head examined.

Regardless of the unintentional backstage comedy, I finally managed to pull my act together. It would have saved me a lot of needless blunders if I'd known then what I know now. I finally got it right for Oscar night when I was presenting with Tom Selleck, in 1983. I went to my friend Norma Kamali for a dress, which was simple and elegant and looked perfectly gorgeous that night, if I do say so myself. The reaction I got in the press the next day was fabulous. My Oscar appearance was the first time I'd been back to Hollywood since my success on Broadway in *Woman of the Year*. It felt like a rite of passage.

I had redeemed my career after the MGM crisis and regained critical respect and public support. The way I carried myself in that dress said it all. I was no longer just the girl in the bikini.

Dressing Down

I've said a lot about dressing up, but very little about dressing down. Come on! Who walks around with every hair in place all the time? Don't neglect dressing for comfort. Put an outfit together on the spur of the moment that is charming, unassuming, and unpretentious. No one likes a stuffed shirt. It's not much fun to be one, either.

Being in the public eye, even during off-hours, can be a drag. I found myself fretting far too much about what to wear, even just to run around town. In my early days I didn't dare go to the corner drugstore without getting dressed to kill. Eventually, I eased up a bit and relaxed. But that doesn't change the fact that I'm always aware I'm going to be noticed.

These days, I don't shop on Madison Avenue or Rodeo Drive or Robertson Boulevard when the paparazzi are out. That's their territory. Also, the streets of Beverly Hills and Manhattan's SoHo are loaded with

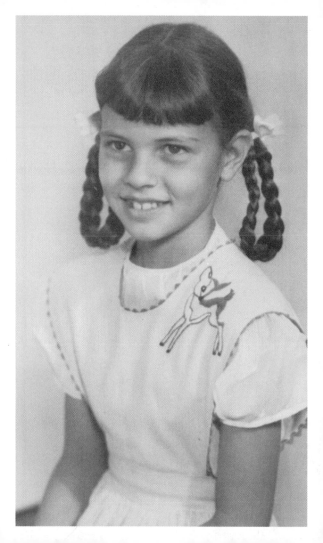

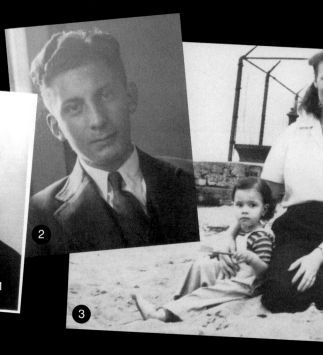

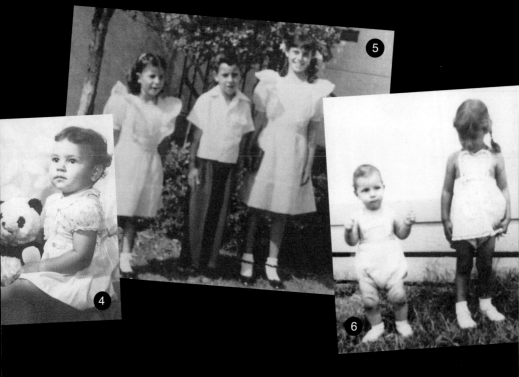

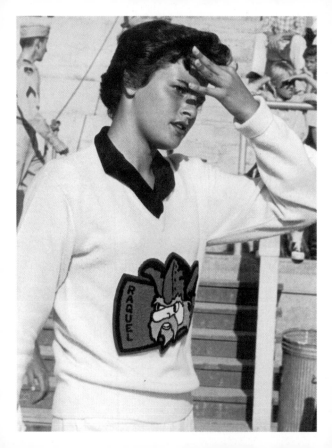

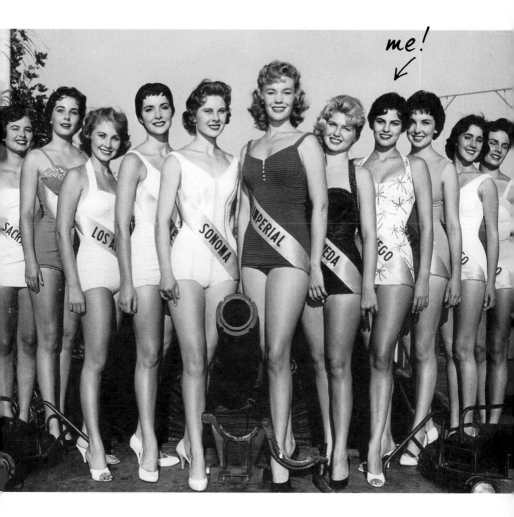

me!

Left: I made cheerleader at 15. Rooting for the La Jolla Vikings!

Above: Beauty contest line-up for the state title - "Maid of California" 1956. (I won.)

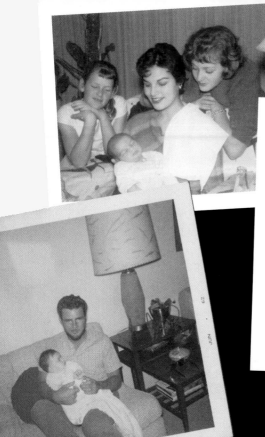

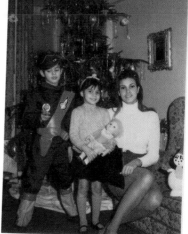

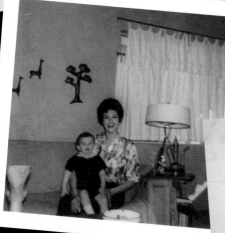

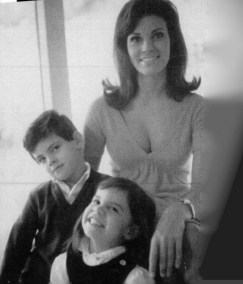

Clockwise from top left:
Newborn son Damon with
Mommy and Aunties Jerri
(left) and Judy (right).
Christmas in London 1965,
with Damon and Tahnee.
Before breaking into movies,
I took a job as a cocktail
waitress complete with toga
and blonde wig! Mommy stylin'
and baby Tahnee, cruisin' 1962.
Jim Welch lookin' sharp in
his uniform – Green Beret.
Our little threesome enjoying
success – courtesy of new
contract with Fox Studios.
Me in beehive hairdo,
with baby Damon in his
first suit! Proud papa Jim,
cradling new daughter,
Tahnee.

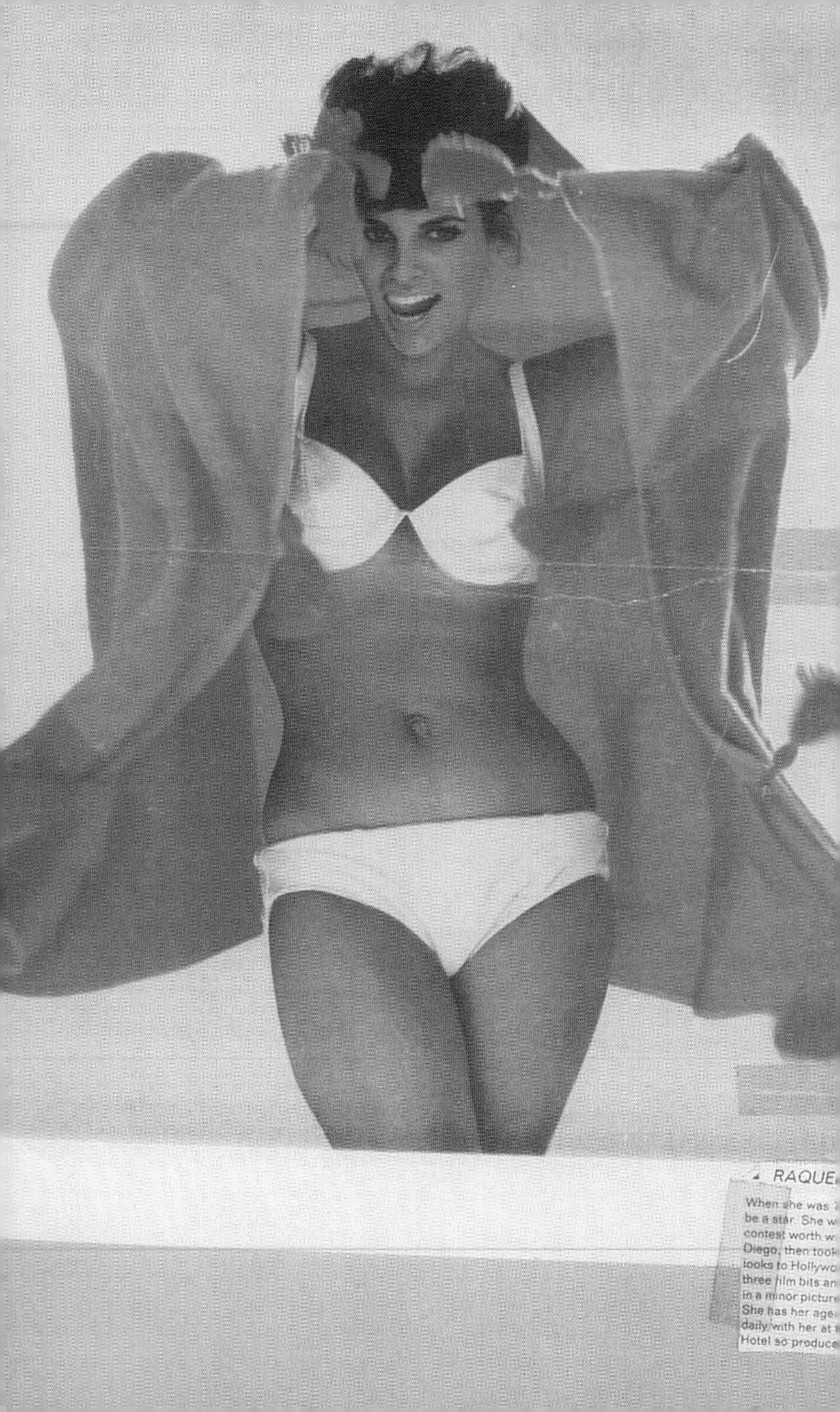
RAQUE
When she was
be a star. She
contest worth
Diego, then took
looks to Hollywo
three film bits an
in a minor pictur
She has her age
daily with her at
Hotel so produce

Left to right clock-
wise: Life magazine
pictorial "The End
of the Great Girl
Drought," jump-
started my career
in 1964. My first
time in a movie,
with Elvis! (Check
the lady-like out-
fit). Adrift in a
dingy using my
watercolor box as
make-up kit.
"Fathom" - 1967.
Loana, Queen of the
Shell People -
turned up on hun-
dreds of magazine
covers - 1966.
Falling for hunky
Stephen Boyd in
"Fantastic Voyage"
- 1964.
Ready for action
with guns 'n' ammo -
"100 Rifles." Bare
midriff, pin-up pose
below.

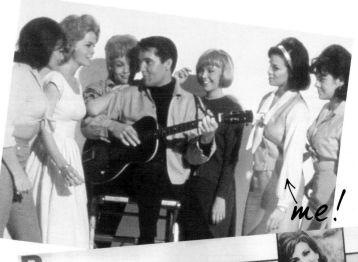

← me!

Raquel on horseback for "100 Rifles"

**Now They've Put
Her on Horseback**

IN HER latest movie, "100
Rifles," Raquel Welch, according to the script, has
to run a mile in a scorching
desert, bounce down a vertical
embankment on a runaway
horse and engage in hand-to-
hand combat with Mexican
soldiers. Director Tom Gries
commented, "I never expected
her to do the stunts herself,
but she insisted and was sen-
sational."

Miss Welch commented,
"People are surprised that I
can do such things, but that's
just because they expect me
to stand still and look sexy."

Just so too many fans won't
be disappointed, there is a
scene in "100 Rifles" where
she strips and showers under
a water tower in front of
a trainload of soldiers. A girl
has to keep clean. Doesn't
she?

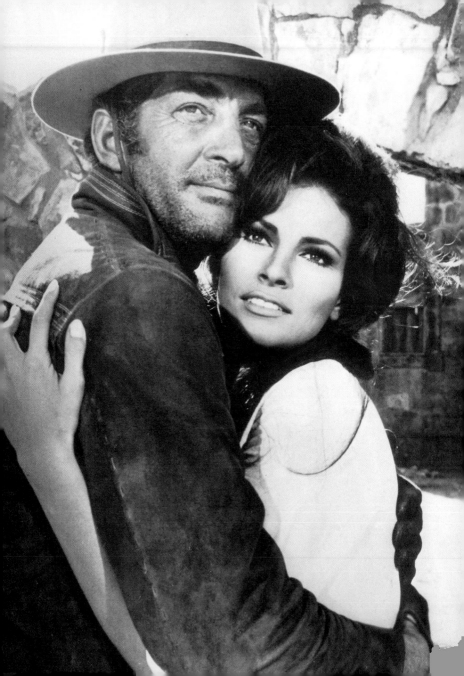

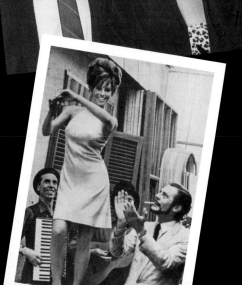

Left to right clockwise:
Embracing Mr. Cool in
"Bandolero" - 1968. Frank and I
palling around off set, "Lady in
Cement" - 1968. Close exchange
with Burt Reynolds in "100
Rifles." With Richard Burton,
backstage at "Woman of the
Year," Palace Theatre - 1983.
Dancing on tabletop with dream-
boat Marcello Mastroianni -
Rome 1966.

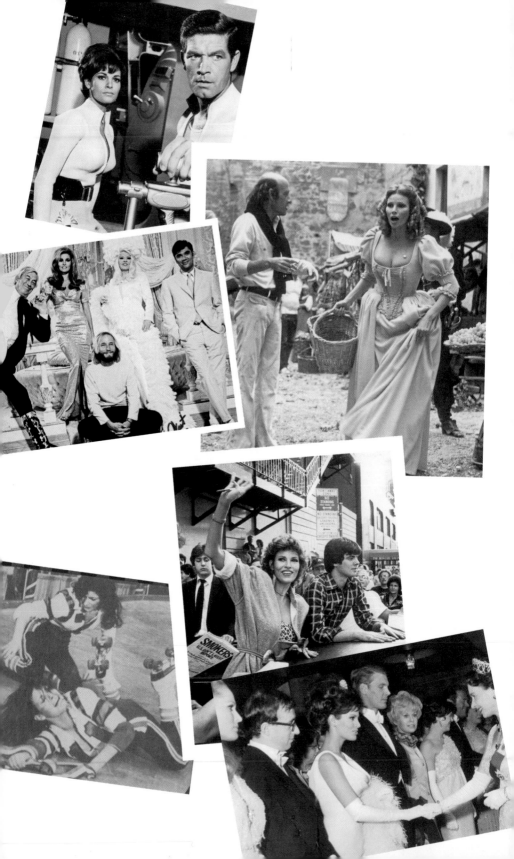

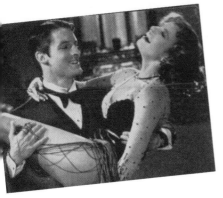

Clockwise from top left:
Playing a marine biologist in
"Fantastic Voyage" with Stephen Boyd.
Both of us upstaged by the cleft in his
chin. Comedy genius, director Dick
Lester, liked to trip me up for laughs on
"Three Musketeers." Carried away by
Perry King in "Wild Party" dance
sequence - 1975. On-stage in B'way
musical "Woman of the Year." Dance
number One of the Boys. 1982-83.
Ursula Andress, Woody Allen, me,
James Fox, and others presented
to the Queen at a Royal Command
Performance - 1966. Damon and I lean
on limo to greet fans and sign
autographs - 1983. Actress Helena
Kallianiotes and I duke-it-out
in roller derby flick, "Kansas City
Bomber" - 1972. (L to R) John
Houston, me, Mae West, and movie
critic Rex Reed were all aboard the
"Myra Breckenridge" train. Director,
Mike Sarne, seated in front.

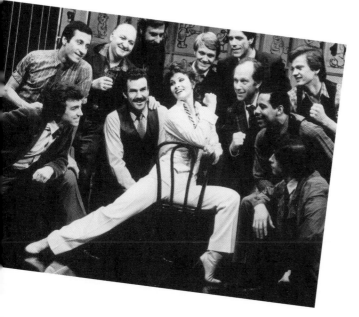

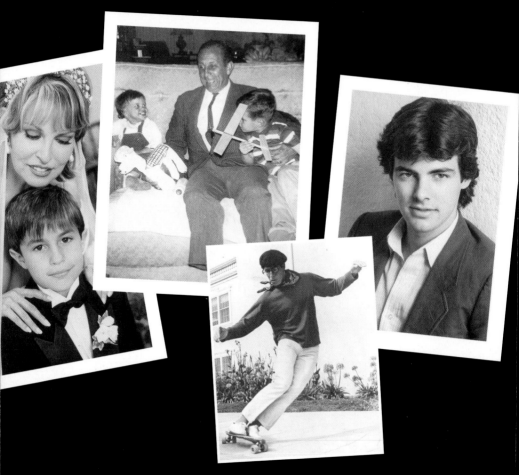

Left to right: My wedding day with adorable Best Man – Little Richie. Grandpa, playing with grandchildren, Tahnee 2, Damon 4. My handsome son Damon . . . Smart with heart. My athletic brother Jim, "Castillo," skateboarding in La Jolla.

Clockwise from tope left: My gorgeous daughter Tahnee . . . Talent and Beauty. My best friend and amazing sister, Gayle –visiting me on film set – 1993.

Making an
entrance wearing
an "almost there"
beaded dress
by Bob Mackie.

tourists hoping to spot someone. In most other neighborhoods, folks aren't expecting anyone famous, so by the time they figure it out, you're gone. The Grove and the Farmers Market in Hollywood can be infested with shutterbugs. This is also true of the Ivy, Mr. Chow's, the Marmont, and other hangouts in H'wood, Santa Monica, and Malibu. Unless you want to be a hermit, the dilemma is, "How can I let my hair down without letting myself go?"

Here's how I approach being incognito. My favorite knock-around uniform these days is a pair of dark navy or black jeans and a T-shirt, with a cool jacket. I always grab a hat and sunglasses. I find that as long as my clothes fit well, even if they're weekend gear, I'll be okay.

If I want to go unnoticed on the streets of New York in fall, I slip into a sweater and pants. I add a trench coat and a scarf, grab my cheese-cutter cap, and I'm out the door. I used to dread the possibility that people would recognize me when I wasn't in movie-star mode, but *they* don't seem to mind. In fact, they're quite polite and friendly. After all, there's a time for heavy-duty glamour and a time to be relaxed and easygoing. You can look charming in your cozy clothes. People will wanna "cozy up" to ya.

I've always had a thing for men's clothes: jackets and uniforms: hats, shirts, ties, vests, wristwatches. You name it. Obviously, since the '60s, women's styles have been heavily influenced by men's apparel. I like the way a masculine touch accentuates a girl's femininity; it can prove to be quite sexy. Men's hats have extra dash on a female face. Dietrich, of course, caused a sensation in the '30s by donning naval-officer whites and men's suits. Uniforms, in particular, have a special message. Their strength and durability can look stunning on a member of the fairer sex. And remember the "reveal" out of the welder's helmet in *Flashdance*? Contrasts make an impact!

For casual wear, I often go scavenging through army surplus shops for authentic flight suits, bomber jackets, etc. They're great for shopping around town, weekends in the country, and short trips to vacation spots. Though they're obviously not for everyone, I always enjoy wearing them, and men seem to get the joke. You have to pick your occasion and know what the traffic will bear. Somehow, I can't picture this kind of getup on the adorable Betty White. But that girl is full of surprises.

Age-Appropriate Dressing

Learning to dress appropriately at any age is an acquired skill that doesn't come naturally for most of us. It develops with practice. Even when a youthful woman makes a fashion faux pas, it can have repercussions that are devastating. The stakes are higher once you pass fifty. It seems there are endless opportunities to make a fool of yourself with each passing year. It's so awfully hard to get it right.

My own faux pas are doubly mortifying because they're sometimes documented in photos. One might hope that as we Golden Girls age, we would be granted some immunity, but there's no free pass. We still can't get away with much.

Indeed, the standards are higher for older women now that we're better preserved than previous generations. Our fashion choices need to be more precise than in younger years, when the glow of youth could lessen any lapse in taste and judgment. Whether it's the length of a skirt, the plunge of a neckline or an unflattering ensemble, dressing becomes an obstacle course the older you get.

American pop culture isn't very sympathetic. It seeks to ridicule every stage of life and turn it into a cliché. For instance, I recently received a video by e-mail in honor of the "50th anniversary of Barbie" . . . who now has morphed into "Cougar Barbie," complete with Botox needles, a stable of young men, and a Wonderbra. When unhooked, the bra drops two saggy boobs to the floor! The whole thing would be hilarious if it didn't impose such an unflattering stereotype of today's older woman. We are so often pictured as grotesque, desperate, artificial, shallow, and downright scary.

A recent skit on *Saturday Night Live* had a stinging parody of women of the boomer generation. We are seen as having no role to play in American society except as sexual predators, masquerading as aging hookers. *SNL* views women over fifty as a bunch of losers.

Unfortunately, the harsh ridicule rings all too true if you take into account the endless string of reality TV shows that focus on women approaching fifty, many of whom seem oblivious to reality. As entertaining as these ladies are to watch, with few exceptions, what they embody doesn't help the cause of women in general. The impression they often leave is of overly superficial, highly competitive, materialistic, catty women, who are obsessed with status and are prone to some pretty unfortunate fashion choices. How do I know this? Because I tune in.

Such shows have produced some questionable role models for the viewing public. Reality clones are cropping up in malls across the country, leaving behind an unflattering picture of what older women are like today. It's too bad the mall ladies don't turn for inspiration to the likes of Helen Mirren. Now, there's a worthy goddess.

A Matter of Good Taste

Mature women should leave certain fashion choices to younger types. We need an AAD program (Age Appropriate Dressing) for women in their fifties and sixties who are addicted to dressing like they're in their twenties. Show a little restraint, ladies. Though you may look good for your age, let's not lose touch with reality. It's far preferable to concentrate on being comfortable in your own skin, and move on with your life.

Part IV

A WOMAN
AND HER
WORLD

TWELVE

Where Do We Go From Here?—Dating

Picking up the Pieces and Moving On

It's over. Where do I go from here? It's a haunting question that resurfaces whenever a relationship has run its course and ended. There must be millions of women who, like me, are recently divorced or widowed, or have broken up and find themselves past fifty and on their own. For me, after the fourth go-round, I felt like a failure; I was angry with myself and *him* and felt a huge wave of sadness wash over me. There is definitely a period of mourning, while the loss of intimacy with your "other half" fades away. But you always carry that sense of loss. The immediate impulse is to cover it up and fill the hole in your heart . . . anything to stop the pain and the endless rehashing of what went wrong: Did he want me to leave? Does that explain his behavior? Was I right to kick him out? Or . . . did I screw up? Why couldn't he open up to me? Damn, those unanswerable questions, along with the endless self-recriminations and second-guessing. And now, I find myself staring numbly into a void.

Whether the relationship crashed and burned or eroded over time, whether he walked out, cheated, or you simply got to the point where you found yourself living with a stranger, is immaterial. It's what comes next that matters. Are we going to repeat the same patterns again out of an urge to move on too quickly? Or is this an opportunity to take a closer look at ourselves and the part our actions and thoughts played in what just happened? Thoughts do lead to actions. Sooner or later, whatever we are thinking about our partner will be demonstrated.

Who am I to talk? After my fourth divorce, I had to ask myself, "Do I want to go for number five?" God knows, I've had enough practice, so maybe next time I'll get it right. And then again, maybe I'm just not a good candidate for marriage. I'll admit that I'm pretty self-involved, as most actresses are, though I'm not proud of it. The men I love often find themselves in competition for my attention with other interests in my life. I try my best to make them feel like they're the *most* important thing to me besides my children (which *is* true), but not the *only* thing that I love. I think that's honest. On the other hand, no matter how much I dote and defer to him, I cannot fill in the blanks in *his* self-esteem all on my own. I wish I could. Even with all the frustration, I still love the company of interesting, attractive men. And yet, to be honest, I'm really not looking. I've grown tired of going down the same road once again, almost by habit. I *could*, of course, change my mind at the drop of a hat. But don't count on it. By now, I know *waaay* too much. And where does it all lead?

Looking ahead, one has to ask, "Will there ever be a time in my life when I can stop appeasing a man and refrain from looking for a reflection of my worth in his eyes?" I personally need a breather from that. For the moment, I prefer my privacy. Perhaps because I'm getting older, there's an urge to streamline and simplify my life. It's a new time, a new world, and I'm looking forward to it. Now is the time when it's important for me to take stock, make amends and deal with regrets.

Women of a certain age need *not* feel compelled to have a man in their lives. I believe if it's meant to be, it will happen. Let life unfold as it will. I would encourage you to enjoy the perks of living alone . . . at least for a significant period of time, and abstain from being desperate. Your friends will no doubt encourage you to date and find someone new. But this feeds into *an obligation to repeat the same patterns — instead of living in the now and exploring something new.* I'm all for the latter. My "now," for example, has turned into a fabulous and productive period that doesn't allow much time to fret over the lack of a man. Where would he fit in? There's a neon sign flashing on and off in my head that reads "No Vacancy."

My time these days is occupied by my friends of both sexes, my colleagues and fellow artists, my darling brother and sister, my two terrific kids, my social and community interests, my church activities, and my professional life, all of which have made for a very full, rich period. I turned the corner after the failure of my last marriage and realized in retrospect that the presence of a man was *not* so essential. Sometimes having a partner is simply masking one's fear of being alone.

I haven't always had the time to experience the sheer joy of living. Year after year I worked my tail off with few chances to catch my breath or pursue a *normal* routine. And now, thank God, I can! It's a real luxury, one that I plan to indulge in to the fullest.

The obvious question is . . . do I miss the sex? Frankly, in marriage, sex really isn't the glue that holds everything together. I can remember only one past relationship in which the sex continued along with the same intoxicating heat that it had at the beginning. Strangely enough, that was the *only* thing that worked in that relationship. Outside the bedroom, we were skating on thin ice. So what exactly *am* I missing? Sex, in my opinion, is overrated and constantly hyped far beyond what it can deliver. Good sex is really the by-product of how the rapport in your relationship is going otherwise. If you're lucky, it occurs with some regularity and becomes an expression of your continuing love for each other. But it's not the whole enchilada. This is a philosophy that I don't expect many will agree with or understand—especially those who will no doubt think I'm a poor soul if I'm not *with* a man. Men are, after all, *indispensable.* If you don't believe it . . . just ask *them!*

Another reason for staying unattached is that I am always busy, and something would have to suffer to make room for a serious commitment. It's been my experience that the demands of a career usually interfere with or interrupt any successful rapport between a man and woman. Think about it . . . Usually, when you're having fabulous sex, including those *looong* weekends, late nights, daily distractions, missing lunch hours, and getaways that extend into guilt-ridden trysts out of town, it all ends on a rather uncomfortable note. While disappearing into a netherworld of bliss, the rest of your life and work takes a nosedive. Yeah, yeah, in the beginning it may be justified and tend to lighten your step, and friends do seem happy for you; but when you finally come up for air, don't be surprised to find that those same people look at you like, "Where in hell have *you* been?" Or worse, everyone has simply moved on . . . without you.

Here's a question for you women out there: Can every man you fancy fit into your life with its professional and private commitments? Or is he going to upset the apple cart and destroy the balance of things? Sound selfish? Maybe. But it's a reality. Is this romantic liaison going to prove to be a positive or destructive influence in your life? And most important of all, is he absolutely worth it? Don't forget, even if you are a bit older, your grown children and extended family have to be on board with the idea. And they're not the only ones who have a vote.

There's also the question of money. Say hello to a popular syndrome, alive and thriving among men today, who attach themselves to women who will "carry" them financially. A man's masculine pride in providing support has morphed into wanting a woman to take care of him like a mommy and, yes, provide for all his financial needs as well. Some of these dudes walk away from a relationship with a big "take." So it's something to think about, especially now that professional women have often built up quite an impressive annuity in later life. *Cau-*

tion: Now is not the time to act like a schoolgirl and choose a partner just because he's eye candy. *Capiche?* Of course, there is the classic prenup agreement, but why get married to someone you cannot trust? No wonder so many professional women are opting to cohabit with a guy out of wedlock. Remind yourself that you are past the childbearing age. It's wise to consider the landscape you will be traveling through before barging ahead in search of an emotional refuge.

We've all heard the popular theory that you have to take risks in order to find love, and to some degree, it's true. And yet, looking back, such risks seem more relevant when you're living the first half of your life, and your youthful biology is clearly timed to procreate. That's when an avalanche of hormones leads us all around by the nose. I can vividly remember feeling a compelling urgency to find a mate. It's no wonder that back in my generation parents always tried so hard to rein us in. Those are the *frisky* years when a girl can get pregnant just by thinking about it. As I mature, I don't feel that overwhelming pull. Instead, I've felt a shift in what I really *want* and a distance between my desires and what I genuinely *need*. It actually feels really good. I guess you could say that I honestly don't sense that I'm missing anything, so I'm not inclined to look further for happiness.

I'm not discounting the fact that I am strongly attracted to certain men and still might nurture a burning desire to be with them. I'll also admit that when it happens, I feel those adolescent hormones raging again, like a teenager. But now it doesn't knock me off balance the way it once did. If things don't work out between us, my world and happiness are not ruined, as they were years ago. I look at it this way: If a partner can really add something special to my life, then it's meant to be. If he is only going to cause a hassle . . . forget about it.

Living Alone and Loving It

Brief backstory: When I was well into my fifties, I suddenly realized that I'd barely spent any time in my life living alone. I'd gotten married to my high school sweetheart, James Wesley Welch, at nineteen. Sadly, just a few years later—after the birth of our two beautiful children—our very young and challenged union didn't last. Following our divorce, I left town and later became involved with a couple of serious boyfriends, neither of whom went the distance. A few years after that (1967), I ended up married for the second time, to Patrick Curtis, whom I met after coming to Hollywood and who insinuated himself, with my tacit consent, into my early career. That relationship fell on rocky footing once I had "made it," but lasted through several of my early films, until it ended in divorce in 1970. This was followed by two consecutive committed relationships, leading up to my French period, when I met my third husband. In 1977, while filming a romantic comedy in Paris with Jean-Paul Belmondo called *L'animal,* I was introduced to a young screenwriter and director, André Weinfeld. He was charming and witty and spoke perfect English. Our courtship and marriage lasted about twelve years.

Just as my relationship with André began to falter, I became acquainted with a very attractive man while filming a movie in Los Angeles, and we began a heated and extended romance. We were together almost 24/7 for approximately six years; but in the end, to put it in his words, "we were from two different worlds." It wasn't a good idea for us to get married. I don't mean to barrel along like a travelogue or to trivialize any of these relationships, but suffice it to say, by the time I started to take stock of my life, I was in my fifties; and I concluded that I desperately needed to carve out some personal time to be on my own. Consequently, instead of letting myself get swept into the arms of yet another man, I deliberately steered clear of any such entanglement. At this point I felt I owed it to myself to learn how to live without all the testosterone overspill. I also had to acknowledge that perhaps in the past I'd been afraid of being a single woman. It was time to change all that. Well, I'm nothing if not up for a new challenge.

My intuition signaled that I'd been actively avoiding a personal crisis, one that involved facing my subconscious thoughts, my deferred (no, buried) feelings and the guilt and regret that was lurking unresolved within me. Men had been a welcome refuge from my innermost thoughts. For me, the act of surrender to a man began to smack of *running away from* the painful doubt that comes with solitude. Like many women, I preferred to lose myself in the gaze of a lover's eyes, rather than face an honest self-appraisal. I needed to stop the role-playing and accept myself, without the camouflage.

And yet, "flying solo" isn't exactly well-received socially. I felt as if I were caught up in a Jane Austen novel, in which a woman is still judged by her male partner, and "marrying up" brings the highest accolades. It's a social conceit that seems to demand compliance far too often. Consequently, I hear the same inquiries over and over again: "Are you dating anyone? Is there a man in your life?" As though this were *the* prerequisite for happiness. Nothing else seems to matter. Nevertheless, I'm at the point when pleasing and impressing others has fallen from the top of my list. I'm not faking it when I say that I enjoy my freedom. I no longer feel the urgent need to be one half of a couple. Which raises the subject of whether the onslaught of menopause could lead to a drop in libido? The answer is yes; however, the effect on sexual desire varies greatly from woman to woman. I can only speak for myself and say that I definitely did not lose my sex drive . . . if anything, it is every bit as responsive as ever. But my mental, psychological, and spiritual side has a more passionate need to be fed than when I was younger, maybe because I often left these demands on the back burner. I have the sense that the biological urgency to procreate eclipsed my other needs for a time. But there is a fine distinction between the "biological clock" demanding to be heard and sexual *desire* continuing into old age.

What's the panic? Men reconnect after a breakup with such lightning speed that you wonder if they're more terrified of being alone than we are. But is it truly necessary to enter into some kind of face-saving competition with your ex, simply for appearance's sake? It smacks to me of high school. Despite my near addiction to men earlier in life, I find that currently I am quite secure on my own. After all, a relationship comes with a mammoth obligation of time and energy. And yet, I wouldn't close the door on the pleasures of falling for someone who resembles, say, Hugh Jackman. Alas, he's too young for me!

Younger Men

It's considered a real coup for a woman of a certain age to be seen on the arm of a younger man. However, what was a rarity only a few decades ago has lately become a trend for only slightly faded women of the boomer generation, who are much better preserved than their mothers and clearly relish the chance to turn the tables on older men and their bimbos. In recent years, there has been a veritable stampede of older women looking to rob the cradles of younger men. Rodeo Drive is rife with well-heeled cougars, primed and ready to pounce. In reality, I don't think bagging a younger dude is much of a challenge when you're still in your forties. As I noted previously, the fourth decade is a cakewalk. Save the kudos for those women in their fifties and beyond who can still turn heads.

It's undeniable that a growing number of older women could qualify as "Golden Babes" and see themselves as the counterpart to attractive older men. But few have turned that fantasy into reality. And not every woman likes the role of predator. Despite my image, I prefer to be pursued rather than take the lead. Careful . . . is the ego boost you get from attracting a younger man just another proving ground to illustrate that you've "still got it"? Are we in danger of kidding ourselves?

Occasionally I've hit it off with a decidedly younger man and haven't wanted to deal with the consequences until later. But as I get older, especially with younger guys, I try to keep the rapport platonic so that neither of us feels pressured or threatened. It's almost unheard-of anymore, but I tend to value a man, regardless of age, for himself, instead of as a means to a *skin fix*, which is how some women refer to a sexual encounter that doesn't involve any emotional attachment. I am not built that way. I prefer to know the man I may or may not become intimate with. My feminine nature demands a chance to relate on a more personal level than just sex, and to develop a comfortable rapport before advancing to the touching stage. I think I'm pretty typical in this regard. It makes the passionate moments better, so there's no need for faking it. The only hiccup is that sometimes you can end up destroying a great long-standing male friendship by letting it graduate to a buddy hump.

Since my thirties, I've been in serious relationships with younger men, and I saw no reason not to be . . . *then*. I met my third husband, André, when I was thirty-seven. Though he was seven years younger than me, the age difference didn't really play into our relationship in any significant way. He didn't seem younger, I suppose because he came off as superintelligent, multitalented, and extremely funny. But it's quite a different story after a woman hits fifty. Après fifty, it's rare to find a much younger man who has the maturity, sophistication, and romantic experience to live up to expectations inside and outside the bedroom. I'm referring to men who have not developed a sexual vocabulary even by their mid-forties. Sad but true. The reasons for this blind spot are complicated, to say the least. Has the gay world siphoned off all the truly sensual men? Are hetero men increasingly intimidated by women? Are the metrosexuals just too *into* themselves? Or are some men focused on women only as trophies, preferring the company of male cronies instead, leaving women aside as objects of desire, a subject they never did very well in to begin with?

A liaison with a younger man of limited aptitude can prove disappointing. Some of the younger men in my life, although they were decidedly sophisticated in other areas, unexpectedly needed a little tutorial in the bedroom. In other words, there was a surprise in store for me behind closed doors when I discovered that they hadn't studied up on the geography of a woman. It happens! If you decide to venture in where wiser heads fear to go, you could wind up becoming a cruise director in the boudoir.

Frustrating as it is, the rule is never to become critical of his performance or make selfish demands. If he's a *keeper* in other ways, tap into the softer side of your nature — if you have one — and give him some time.

He'll likely come around if you have patience and allow him to feel like he is *the* lover you want to be with and not a failure in that department.

I'm told that it takes guts for a man to approach a famous woman. If he's younger, the stress factor could edge up a notch or two. I wouldn't know what he's going through at that point, but I can attest to the fact that if and when things progress to the point of consummating the relationship, the pressure mounts still more on *his* end. He may be prone to drink just a little too much . . . and, well, I've been there . . . haven't you? That pretty much stops things cold. And then what? Well, you can toss him out or give him a chance to grow in confidence . . . and in other areas, too. But seriously, it takes two people in sync to make the physical part lift off. Sometimes you can't expect to hit the high notes without a little rehearsal. You may have to subtly teach him a thing or two. Who knows; he may turn out to be a quick study!

Not every single younger guy needs diapering, but there are a number of other areas besides sex where you might be more knowledgeable than he is; for example, business, social networking, and juggling lifestyles. No wonder Marilyn Monroe, who was wicked smart, sugarcoated everything. A smart woman may have an analytical edge that *could* help her partner with pending business decisions or negotiations, which are, traditionally, *a man's domain*. You may spot the liabilities inherent in his investments or see the implications in his interactions with friends and colleagues, but you might have to stifle yourself until he decides to *ask* for your opinion. He probably needs to prove himself capable in your eyes. So step lightly, at your own risk. Such tendencies are the case with most men, regardless of age. Men don't like to be made aware that a woman knows as much or more than they do. He may even pull away. If he should falter in his profession or lose his job . . . he's going to feel like he's lost face. And then forget about the sex.

Your level of compatibility as a couple outside the bedroom affects what happens behind closed doors, and vice versa. You cannot compartmentalize your intimate relationship from the rest of your life. When problems do arise, try not to be the one to find fault. If he *does* turn to you, *suggest*, but don't *tell*, him what to do, and keep it brief. What's the point of rehashing where he went wrong? Let *him* say he wants to change or alter things. Come up with an alternate idea that he can consider. Many men seem to remain little boys forever; but when a woman reaches adulthood, she tends to weigh things more carefully. She's not afraid to meditate, pray, seek counsel, or even enroll in a Twelve-Step program if it will help. Women trust that the solution is out there, given a chance to present itself in an atmosphere of love and trust. I believe that behind every successful man is a strong, caring woman, be she a mother, a wife, or a life partner. She has to be willing to let him shine.

But where, oh where can we women go, when *we* need support and sound advice? I prefer to go to my man and ask for his opinion and guidance. I want to bounce ideas off him and get his take on things. I want to feel protected. What if you don't genuinely respect your partner's character and choices? Then what? Perhaps it's time to ask yourself if you are with him primarily because he's your boy toy. If the answer is yes, then he's been miscast, and that alone could kill it for you. Being with a younger man might not be all it's cracked up to be. In some ways it gives *you* the upper hand; and you may prefer it that way. But there are those women — myself among them — who would much prefer that the relationship be more balanced.

Keeping Up with Him

What about keeping up with a younger guy? Is the age difference going to be a problem? For one thing, there is a stamina difference between men and women, regardless of age. I don't think it need be cause for concern, though there have been times when I just wanted to roll over and play dead after a night on the town. Usually, I like to pace myself when scheduling my day or my calendar, knowing that I need a little time to "gas up" before jumping back into the swim of things. In fairness, I was always that way, even in my twenties, but now I don't push myself so hard. If he's looking for a party animal, you gotta ask yourself if you're really up for that. Maybe . . . not so much?

Overall, I think it's fairly safe to say that most men realize from the example of their mothers and sisters that women are more high maintenance. They accept that women have an epic prep time for special occasions. But on an *everyday basis*, they expect their lady to be more spontaneous. I've found a girl needs to be able to roll with the tide and make adjustments. We've all gotten up earlier to make breakfast and be there for him, to see him off, or accompany him to the gym. There are also times when you need to be low maintenance and able to pick up and go. You have to be versatile, like his sports car, with different gears and speeds. On the other hand, I've also noticed that most men will accommodate my natural pace on the weekends.

It's not necessary to move through life like conjoined twins. In the early stages of the mating game, being inseparable might be a compulsion, but further down the line, both parties need their space. Generally speaking, men and women move at different speeds, but it depends on the guy. As I see it, it's not really a question of age. It's a question of thoughtful consideration. So count backward from blastoff to give yourself reasonable time to do your thing. And, when you reappear, make him feel you're worth waiting for. Just let him know in advance *when* you'll be ready and stick to it . . . men hate to be kept waiting.

Are you into sports? Are you ready for an afternoon of car shows, the Super Bowl game, the Lakers, the World Series, or the World Cup? You know the drill. If you don't like sports and he's a rabid fan, it's going to be a drag for one of you. I happen to love football, soccer, baseball, basketball, hockey, plus boxing, tennis, and golf as spectator sports. But if your fella is really athletic and likes to participate in any of these sports, including skiing, surfing, or sailing, etc., then I hope you will also enjoy one or more of these activities and can join in the fun.

Fortunately, with few exceptions, most men have sports buddies who accompany them for such activities and outings, leaving you free to do your own thing while he spends time with the boys; and there's nothing wrong with that. In fact, it's a good thing. Everyone needs an opportunity to bond with pals and blow off steam. But this raises the question of exactly who his friends are and what kind of unsavory habits and skirt-chasing tendencies they bring into the mix. That's another story, and yet a reminder that it's not him alone you'll be involved with; it's his whole world. In fact, in many cases, stamina is less of a problem than finding common tastes and interests.

During the summer months, if Mr. Stud Muffin is a boat guy, then you're in for a ride. Boating requires planning, and you'll need to clear some time for packing and shopping for boat supplies, then spending the entire day or longer aboard a boat . . . especially if it's a holiday weekend. Of course, if we're talking a yacht with a full crew and chef, then you just need to arrive with a tan and several changes of swimsuits. But don't even sign up if you don't like being out on the water and are prone to seasickness . . . 'cause a sailor is a beer-swilling rogue with no sense of what day it is, and those patches and Dramamine tablets only go so far. You are in Jimmy Buffettville now!

The biggest fear when dating a younger man is whether you can hold on to him. In the back of every woman's mind is the threat of the "other" woman. If you're an older woman, even a well-preserved one, that threat comes in the form of a younger woman. It goes without saying that you have to stay in shape, but to what extent? Can you realistically compete? I don't think so. You might be prone to blame your age for imagined slights. After all, men will always sneak a peek when they think you're not paying attention. So don't allow yourself to overreact unless it's blatant and disrespectful. As long as he's not engaged in a "come-on" and being openly flirtatious, you're best to remain cool. In truth, don't you, too, like to sneak a peek at handsome men in tight jeans? But his behavior toward you in public says a lot. If he cannot exercise any self-restraint, it doesn't augur well. Any guy who has a chronic roving eye is bound to be a liability.

The bottom line is, what difference does it make whether he becomes interested in a *younger* woman or one *closer to your age*? In both cases, the important thing is to come to grips with the fact that *"he's just*

not that into you!" as demonstrated in the popular chick flick of that title. I would avoid getting involved with a much younger man to begin
with if the main attraction is that he's arm candy and makes you look
good. It could backfire right in your face. And if you are feeling overly
self-conscious in the company of a younger man, then you'd better keep
looking—he's not for you. But he's not to blame for making you feel old.
Only you can do that.

Issues of self-esteem are probably the main thing you'll be dealing with when an age difference is involved. Your feelings can play
tricks on you and rattle your confidence. If *he's* really causing you to feel
not good enough, then what's the point of sticking around? But if it's
in *your own mind*, you can't blame him for confirming what you already
think of yourself. Either way, is this underlying emotional pressure
something you can deal with continually? Know when to walk away.
It's like a miniskirt on a woman past fifty. Even if she's got the legs for
it . . . it's a style better left on the hanger.

Frankly, I have to admit that in spite of the drawbacks, I *am* attracted to younger men; and the feeling, so far, is mutual. But then again,
I haven't had any recent experiences with a man my own age . . . someone in his sixties. I haven't ruled out being with a man who is my contemporary; but to be frank, the good ones are already taken. And if not,
doesn't it seem as if, the older the man, the more he gravitates to girls
thirty years his junior? So there you have it. The fact that youngish men
do actively pursue women in the cougar set makes it easier to ignore the
lack of age-appropriate men for older women.

Did you ever consider that, if the man in your life is more than a
decade younger, he might be faced with taking care of you at some point
in the future? That thought never entered my mind until my mother
passed away. When she died, at ninety-two, she was fortunate enough
to be married to a man thirteen years her junior! To his credit, when
she started to have health issues, he rose to the occasion with flying colors. He surprised us all with how thoughtful and caring he was toward
her when she was failing. He used to brush her hair, give her a bath,
dress her, and even put on her makeup! What a big-hearted senior dude

he turned out to be! He took care of her every need right up to the bitter end. By comparison, I started to realize that the man in my life was quite incapable of stepping up to the plate if anything worse than a runny nose should ever befall me. He acted like he was allergic to such things. Did he have a weak stomach, a weakness in character, or simply a lack of maturity? In fairness, even family may find it difficult to face certain unpleasantness when health issues arise. I guess that's why the marriage vows always *used to* say "in sickness and in health." Is the man in your life capable of keeping that commitment? Are you?

Back in the Dating Pool!

Imagine for a moment that the perfect man is lurking somewhere under the radar. If he's outside your immediate circle, it's not going to be a snap to find him and make a connection. Most people meet someone in the workplace or at college or university. But for many boomers it may be too late for those avenues. Your work life is usually less constant now and often does not include leaving home and joining a "family" of coworkers. So your possibilities for meeting someone lessen drastically. You'd practically have to go on safari in order to sight an eligible bachelor, let alone capture such an exotic creature. Before you start getting your inoculations and cleaning your rifle, you might want to ask yourself if you're really up for such an ambitious expedition. However, if that's what your heart desires, grab your pith helmet and let's forge ahead into the singles jungle for boomers.

Dating? What a concept! If you think you can jump back into the swing of things just like that, you're headed for a rude awakening. It's actually quite shocking how things have changed . . . and I'm not speaking of your waistline. When I started dating again in my mid-fifties, I certainly wasn't prepared for what was in store for me. Before I even got started, some ominous warning signs appeared. Time warp, Raquel! You haven't been dating in *how* many years? I suddenly realized it had been close to eighteen . . . *Eighteen!*

Contrary to what you might expect, I'm not much good at dating. In younger days I must have broken every rule in the book, but now I know better. Perhaps some rules are meant to be broken, but I still have a fondness for certain tried-and-true codes of behavior for dating. I believe they exist to help us avoid a long list of painful mistakes and steer us clear of trouble. Call me crazy and backward, but human history shows that when it comes to the opposite sex, we are often incapable of predicting the long-term consequences of our actions. The plus side of age is that by now we've watched those chickens come home to roost. And yet, even grown women, who should know better, are prone to breaking all the rules and might allow themselves to get caught up in the heat of the moment, once the dance begins. Will we ever learn to act our age? Since when did stupidity become an aphrodisiac?

Anyhow, with my upbringing, I always believed that men were entitled to pursue women, and if they got rejected, fine. Women should never swim out to the wave, so to speak. We can certainly flirt, give off signals, and drop clues, but a woman shouldn't actually pick up the phone and *call* a man. Let him make the first move. Give him time to work up his courage. If you take the lead from the very get-go and he takes the bait . . . look out! Now the stage is set for you to take on the role of instigator and for him to follow. Strong professional women tend to feel they can assume this role without peril. Down the road, when he feels his masculinity dwindle in a million subtle ways, he'll grow to resent you for it.

The beginning of any relationship is rife with missteps and ignored clues. Looking back to precisely the time when you first met *him*, didn't you *know* right off the bat, by instinct, what he was all about? Didn't you hear alarms going off in your head? You knew, didn't you, exactly how everything would turn out? If we're honest with ourselves, we always know. But we don't like to listen. And we've all been guilty of pushing aside our instincts and going full speed ahead. Foolish? Of course. Understandable? Absolutely. Did I care at all about the calamity awaiting me? *Naaah!* I was having too much fun! I probably *could* have avoided some prickly consequences, but who knows? Might I have changed the course of things by not hurling myself from the plane without a 'chute? Maybe. But skydiving is such a thrill!

I myself am timid about making the first move. It doesn't come naturally to me. It also doesn't help that some men are too intimidated to even approach me. In some ways, being famous makes it harder. Nevertheless, I prefer to wait for a guy to act like a man! If he can't work up the courage for that, he's probably not right for me. Yes, it's true; I want the guy to lead. I run my own corporation, for God's sake; I make my own decisions; I'm strong-minded, but . . . there's a limit. I start shrinking back and shuffling around in uncertainty when it comes to "pushing" myself at a man. It takes me forever to work up the moxie to say something, and then, as if by magic, I appear to be very self-possessed. I find it odd that I'm sometimes cast in roles where I appear very "knowing," when the opposite is true. I've even heard people refer to me as a dominatrix, and I understand where that comes from, given some of my film roles. The truth is, the real reason I became an actress was to pretend to be someone else. Rita Hayworth famously lamented, "Every man I have ever known has fallen in love with Gilda and awakened with me." That pretty much says it all.

Who can be Raquel Welch 24/7? Humor helps a lot to get over the image hurdle, when you're me. I love to spar in conversation with an attractive, witty man. A good sense of humor is a real turn-on. Actually, as far as younger men are concerned, it's often better to just keep things light and friendly. Why spoil the rapport between us with the possibility of disappointment? But enough procrastinating! Since I'd been out of the loop for a while, I needed to get myself up to speed on a whole new world of dating!

I had girlfriends who had met guys on the Internet, but I'm not exactly an anonymous face, so that's not for me. Can you imagine? The other thing I realized is that most of the single guys were typically miles younger. That made me quite uncomfortable. Younger guys exude an unsettling aura of trouble. But damn, the idea of a younger man *is* intriguing.

A tale from the trenches: When I least expected it, along came this dude, a Wall Street type, and after some persistence on his part to make a date, I thought, *Where's the harm in it?* He pursued me over the course of several months, during which I was rehearsing a Broadway musical and not available to start something new; and then, in a moment of weakness spiked by my curiosity, I accepted an invitation to go out to dinner with him. No biggie. The catch was, I didn't know this guy very well. He had shown up from out of town at a charity auction in L.A. and bid on a photograph of me. In his mind, a winning bid entitled him to be introduced to me. And now he was following up on that first encounter. *Hmmm.* Can't fault him for trying.

I was bored to tears with showbiz types, and maybe he *would* be interesting. Plus I'd be protected, in my bodyguard-*cum*-chauffer-driven car . . . so, no sweat there.

Have you ever dated someone you're not acquainted with? Even a blind date knows *somebody* whom you know, right? Well, Mr. X and I had only one mutual friend, who called me to vouch for him. But what if this guy, who had the royal chutzpah to ask me out in the first place, turned out to be a no-goodnik? Where was the incentive for him to behave himself? He might reel me in and then what? This was definitely an occasion to tread lightly through the quicksand of "what if's." There was a hint of danger and adventure about the situation. My instincts told me he wasn't a stalker type . . . but that's all I knew. Tall, well-dressed, buttoned-down, polite, and yet—how can I put this?—he was subtly aggressive. *Hmmm, again.*

Oh, did I mention that he was actually *much* younger? Well, he was . . . *twenty years younger!* And here I was entering the open market woefully unprepared; based on preliminary girl talk with my younger friends at the theater, I was ready to throw in the towel. They started coaching me on the latest dating customs, insisting that I carry condoms, and casually rattling off a list of various colors, flavors, and special features available within any city block! Whoa! This caught me completely off guard. You gotta be kiddin' me! What planet am I living on? Do *they* really stash condoms in their purse on a first date? I went to high school in the '50s, and we didn't do that! What's more, I hadn't been playing the field since AIDS had become a major concern. And even before, I had only been in committed relationships. I'm very selective and just don't screw around; in fact, I'd never used a *condumb* — as I like to call them — in my entire life.

Clearly, I was not ready to jump aboard the dating train. I mean, even setting aside the very real threat of STDs, what made anyone think I would go to bed with him the very first night? This was a fast and loose world that I was about to enter and I wasn't inclined to change my modus operandi to fall in line with the new permissiveness. How do girls in their twenties and thirties manage? It's amazing what peer pressure can make you do. Was it *possible* that these younger cuties didn't even *know* that there was another way? But it wasn't just them; many of my contemporaries had become more open to a fling. My friend Charlene, who was a good-time gal and my makeup artist for many years, used to tease me when we were away shooting on location that I was in danger of letting my physical assets go to waste. In her opinion, I wasn't getting enough mileage out of my famous body. "Why dontcha lend it to me for the night?" she asked. "I'll put it to good use!"

So by the eve of my dinner with Mr. New Guy, I was getting cold feet. To quell my nerves, I rationalized that maybe because of *who* I am and because of the fact that I was in NYC doing a musical, he might just want to get to know me socially. Which would be okay. So what was I worried about? He had a good position at a reputable firm; how bad could he be? I mean, I had to date normal guys once in a while, right? Then, just as I had gotten my head together, my young hairdresser slipped me a bag of condoms! "Have fun!" she chirped. *Puhleeze!*

Was I *that* out of touch? Maybe I was too prudish to date anymore? And this guy *was* so much younger, was it possible he thought that I'd have sex with him on the first date? I didn't want to get myself into one of those wrestling matches or some ridiculous, embarrassing situation. Then again . . . what if I *liked* him? That could cause even more trouble. According to my streetwise girlfriends, "If you decide you're really into a guy, he *has to* get a blood test for STDs. He could have AIDS or herpes or warts, or whatever . . ." What a turnoff!

I was, of course, very aware of AIDS by the early '80s when I lost close friends who suddenly became ill and died prematurely. But it had never occurred to me that *I* might have to cope with this problem, given my monogamous history. Now, unfortunately, it had become a fact of life. This was enough to stop anyone cold, but I'd already come this far.

So my date, let's call him Tall, and I headed off to a glamorous restaurant crowded with people, while the car waited curbside to take me back to my apartment afterward, as planned. That would be it: "Good night." But Tall turned out to be both charming and nonthreatening . . . and I dropped my guard. Just as we were getting in the car, he said, "It's a shame to waste such a beautiful evening. Why don't we walk?" He was right about that. The night was warm and balmy, and I was feeling no pain. So we began to stroll along . . . and he took my hand. Tall was lavishing me with compliments, and I got the feeling he was setting me up for "a move." In a lighthearted way, I tried to deflect what seemed to be a come-on. The conversation went something like this:

> ME [*smiling*] You're wasting your smooth talk on me. Shouldn't you be courting my daughter? She's more age-appropriate for you.

> TALL [*laughing*] I'm not interested in your daughter.

> ME You've never met my daughter. She's absolutely gorgeous. You may not be her type, but that's who you should be coming on to. Frankly, I'm old enough to be your *mother*!

I just laid it right out there. As we continued walking, something quite unexpected happened. It was right out of *Sex and the City*. Somehow my high heel broke off on the pavement. Without missing a beat, Tall picked me up and began carrying me down Sixth Avenue, at two o'clock in the morning. There I was, pressed up against him for the whole six blocks to my apartment! And to tell you the truth, I was feeling pretty damn good! I was very conscious of his well-muscled arms. Nice guns! I could feel my defenses crumbling.

But the spell was almost broken when we arrived at my building. I panicked at the sight of the doorman and other attendants in the lobby. Remember, I'm a California girl, and we're not used to doormen and the like. We live in houses, not condos. So now, the doorman is in on my personal moment with Tall, as are the freakin' desk guy and the elevator operator. They *all* know! It'll spread like wildfire through the building. What's to stop any one of them from picking up the phone to Page Six?

I was feeling very awkward, but Tall put me down smack in the middle of the lobby and without warning, laid one mind-blowing kiss on me . . . and I was thinking, "Damn, he's hot!" Suddenly I didn't want to pass him on to my daughter. And a voice in my head said, "You can carry this off, Rocky, you still look good . . ."

Tall had promise. It *was* a memorable first date, but the whole thing fizzled. So much for the power of a first kiss. It was sad, but I had to break it off.

Fortunately, the safety brakes on my libido were in working order, though they seemed a bit rusty at first. With a fair share of resolve, my runaway emotions skidded to a halt and I was saved from a crash landing. That was too close for comfort.

Famous Men

I don't want to inspire envy in the hearts of my female fans, but it seems odd not to mention that over the years my dating pool has often included some of the most desirable men on the planet. How lucky can you get? I'd be lying if I didn't admit that on occasion I was susceptible to their charms. After all, I was working with and had friendships with some extraordinary men. Among them were movie stars, sports heroes, music legends, business tycoons, and moguls. Being in their company was always exhilarating and stimulating. In some cases it went beyond mere acquaintance, but because of the fame factor, that's a private matter.

I'm only human, so of course I found myself in situations where the air was charged with sexual electricity, and I ended up "seeing" some of these well-known heartthrobs undercover. But boy, I tried to avoid waking up to the smell of paparazzi in the morning just before heading out for breakfast. Nor do I like it when room service gives away my room number or snitches on which entrance *we* are leaving from. It just kills the whole damn thing. That's where fame takes its toll.

I'm not the kiss-and-tell kind, but to save you racking your brain over which of my leading men I spent personal time with, I'll narrow it down for you. Let's see if you can guess which ones made me weak in the knees. Was it Dean Martin, Frank Sinatra, Elvis, or Stephen Boyd? Burt Reynolds, Ian McShane, or Richard Burton? Or was it Warren Beatty, Steve McQueen, Dudley Moore, or Marcello Mastroianni, Joe Namath, Tom Jones, Jean-Paul Belmondo, or Oliver Reed? What about Alice Cooper, Burt Bacharach, and Bob Dylan? There were only a few of these guys that I couldn't resist.

Without getting into territory that's too personal, I would say that Dino was very laid back. He was the epitome of cool and had a way of making you come to him. Frank, on the other hand, had a charismatic charm that could knock your socks off. He had a great sense of mischief and took his fun very seriously. Burt Reynolds has a wicked sense of humor. He is street smart and razor sharp but incredibly sweet and even protective with the people he cares about. Richard Burton was like a heat-seeking missile, a smokin' hot romantic. Stephen Boyd had that soft Irish brogue and that cleft in his chin. He had an ironic way of looking at things and a witty charm about him. Elvis was like high-octane energy, set on idle. He was on hold waiting to be ignited. Dylan is an enigmatic genius, with no need to impress. He doesn't want to be the focus. He's busy observing and sizing it all up. He saves what he has to say for his songs. Burt Bacharach exudes a boyish charm, with a serious perfectionism underneath. He's mellow. Tom Jones is a powerhouse. His vocals will pin you to the wall. They all had that extra something that was like a magnet.

What was remarkable about each and every one of these men was that special aura often referred to as the "sweet smell of success." And for the most part, they were deserving of their accolades. With few exceptions, they all possessed wit, charm, and good looks and were absolutely dripping with charisma . . . and they knew it. It was intoxicating to be around them. Although I found myself attracted to a number of these men, I also found it hard to imagine myself fitting into their world. And believe me, they had a world.

I have a theory that, with few exceptions, such as Elizabeth Taylor and Richard Burton or Brad Pitt and Angelina Jolie, it's hard to make a go of it with the demands of two careers and two egos in the mix. I found that it's pretty damn difficult to nurture an intimate relationship in the glare of the public eye, especially with demanding schedules, long absences that challenge fidelity, the ever-present posse, and the constant eruption of flash bulbs.

It seems that many powerful personalities need an entourage or support system. They include one or more personal assistants, nannies, trainers, makeup artists, hairstylists, fashion stylists, dialogue coaches, chiropractors, cooks and bottle washers, all of whom, believe it or not, have practical reasons to be there. Many male stars simply don't like traveling without their posse. They have an entourage of friends who double as assistants and sometimes a buddy or two they can joke around with during the inevitable downtime that comes with the *hurry up and wait* periods in the movie and entertainment business. His sidekicks are there basically to keep his batteries charged until the moment when he is called into action and ready to *let loose* onstage or on camera. I can't blame these men. To the public, it may seem like an affectation, but I can understand why a guy (or a diva) who performs almost nightly to a live audience needs to keep the adrenaline flowing. The same is true for film work. It's as though he (or she) has to keep the skillet on simmer until ready to serve. People like Elvis, Sinatra, or even Judy Garland lived in a world of their own making. It was either that, or the tendency for a gifted performer seasoned by fame to be a loner and keep to him- or herself. Either way, it doesn't leave much room for anyone else.

And so, without disparaging the lifestyles of the wildly attractive stars I've been close to, I can say that what seems desirable from afar, on closer inspection may not be the right fit. It would be more fun to say that despite everything, the flames of desire exploded into a torrid, scorching affair that swept all reason aside. But my lips are sealed . . . so you choose the ending. Though deep down I knew better, sometimes even I became confused about how I felt. Everyone else seemed so excited and invested in the outcome of a famous liaison that I started to ask myself, "Am I truly attracted to *him* or has he become more of a trophy that others have a stake in?" Should a person get involved solely because of a famous name, like some dingbat groupie? I can relate to that question, because I get completely turned off myself if I suspect that a guy is coming on to me because I'm a status symbol and he can hardly wait to tell his friends.

For me, a man's character is the most important thing about him. It trumps his star status, the size of his bank account, or his studly reputation. If I can't personally feel a genuine attraction to him, then it's a wrap for me. And don't be deluded; powerful men do like to move *faaast*. Some A-list eligible hunks, while being very well-behaved otherwise, *do* feel a sense of entitlement . . . if ya know what I mean. They tend to tear open the package before taking note of the sender. For me, famous or not, it takes some time to get to know someone and ignite that spark.

The disarming reality is that often there's a disconnect between someone's public persona and his off-hours self. There were occasions when I became close to a famous male star but didn't feel a powerful chemistry with the real person behind the bigger-than-life image. The first time it happened, my initial impulse was to wonder, *What's wrong with me?* Aren't I supposed to be feeling something more? Everybody *else* is gaga over this guy. Then comes the realization that the misconceptions you have about someone famous can get in the way. When that happens, it reminds me of my own battle with certain stereotypes that follow me even into my private life. It's not always an easy road to walk.

The takeaway is, whether he's younger, older, famous, successful, or a regular guy, there's no guarantee that it'll be easy. Everyone has their share of problems, as can be witnessed in today's tabloids. It's like catching lightning in a bottle to stumble upon a partner you can really connect with on all levels. But don't buy into the idea that simply because you're older now, there's no chance for you to find happiness with the right man. Just remind yourself, it's a tough market for everyone.

THIRTEEN

Family and Friends

THOUGH WE TEND TO CONCENTRATE ON men and romance in younger days, later down the road it becomes abundantly clear that other relationships like those with family, friends, and coworkers play an equal if not more important role in our lives. Maybe your parents are no longer living. Check. I sure miss mine. Maybe now you're a grandmother. I haven't had that pleasure.

But now, more than ever before, friends have become our extended family. We share our confidences with them, go out shopping and to concerts and the theater with them, and sometimes off on vacation. We invest our time with them and keep them close. We fall in love a little with our close friends and their ways and include them as an indispensable part of our daily existence.

Though any way you look at it, there comes a point where you're faced with reevaluating your pivotal relationships, especially ones with family. Because when we look back—we are reminded that patching up differences, making amends for past wrongs and healing old wounds are now one of the most important things to address with loved ones—before it's too late. There's still so much life left to live; why carry the burden of unresolved personal problems into the future? We all have debts of conscience to pay, and some have nothing to do with mortgages or money.

Reconnecting

I am fortunate enough to have a wonderful brother and sister, who are close to me. Though I haven't spoken much about them, they have become an important part of my life in the past ten years. After we finished school, we all seemed to go our separate ways. I traveled abroad a lot so there were long periods when we connected mainly on birthdays and holidays. You know how that goes. But growing up, we always looked out for one another, and still do.

Exactly two years after I was born, to the day and the month, Mom gave Dad the son he'd been waiting for: my wonderful brother, James Stanford Tejada. We call him Jim. An adorable baby sister, Gayle Carole Tejada, came next; she's three years my junior. What a doll she was! Gayle had the best disposition imaginable. Jim, on the other hand, used to punch me in the stomach when we jockeyed over who could get closest to the floor heater in the winter.

When I was twelve and Gayle was only nine, we began to share a bedroom and a double bed together. Jim slept in the den. I don't know how she lived through my tossing and turning and leg flinging, but she always slept through everything like a log. In general she was very self-contained and always traveled to the beat of her own drum. I think I took up more than my share of the space outside of bed, too, and sometimes it was hard on her. But she never acted like it bothered her.

My getting married at nineteen cut short the bonding time Gayle and I might have had as young women. We didn't really get a chance to continue it until decades later, when Mom's health started to fail. In the '80s, when Gayle, Jim, and I reunited to help Mom, it planted the seeds of what was to come. Over time, the intimacy of our shared experiences wove all our lives back together again. Aside from my children, my beautiful sister Gayle is now my very best friend. Jim travels a lot, but we keep in touch, and there's a bond there between brother and sister Virgos. In fact, we're all more like a family now than when we were kids. Family is everything. Though we went through some rough patches together, it sure was worth it. In the end, my sister and my brother became my soul mates.

Looking Back

When you find yourself suddenly slipping into the role of the older generation, it's almost impossible not to reflect on the past and reassess your life from a new perspective. Because I have few regrets about my love life, I've also come to treasure my single state. I guess the pleasure I take in being self-reliant makes it somewhat easier for me than it is for some women to be unattached and alone. I've noticed that in some ways I think like a man, but at heart, I'm a woman.

I suppose that being the firstborn has something to do with all this. Papa was hoping for a son to carry on the family name but got me instead. He ended up projecting all his hopes and dreams onto my slim shoulders. This didn't make me masculine per se, but it sure had something to do with my drive and ambition. Trying to appease my father, and then, eventually, learning to stand up to him, led me to develop a very strong-minded sense of independence. It gave me the basis to pursue my own career goals rather than allow a man to deny me that choice. Nowadays that inner strength may be what feeds my ability to live happily alone and take pride in being my own person.

Of course, as you already know, Papa caused a lot of conflict in me. Wrapped around that bullet-hard center at my core is an undeniable female sensitivity. Although there are times when I feel like the more fragile feminine side of my nature is being dragged around by the hair. It hurts like hell!

People pay lip service to learning from their mistakes; so now that you've gathered some wisdom along the way, why not use that insight to improve your relationships. In the case of my parents, I would have liked to clear the air and resolve past rifts. I wanted the answers to some gnawing questions, and one more chance to express my love and gratitude before it was too late. I also had hoped that my father would enter his old age without feeling so estranged from the rest of us. There were so many things I was never able to accomplish.

I was floored when my father passed away prematurely. It happened in the intensive care unit, after prostate surgery and was a premature death that could have been avoided. He was only sixty-four! His death was caused by negligence on the part of the hospital, which they admitted the first moment we three kids arrived in the director's office. It took a while before I was able to absorb that I would never see him again.

My father's untimely death brought up a whole truckload of surprising feelings. I was the only family member besides his second wife, Inez, who came to the funeral. My mom, sister and brother didn't attend, so I stood by myself through the brief ceremony. My father's death left an emptiness in me. I didn't know what to do with myself, now that he was gone. It felt odd that I wouldn't have Daddy's expectations to live up to anymore and I was temporarily under the impression that the monkey on my back concerning the daddy issue was gone. Wrong! So after a difficult mourning period, I flew to Brazil to try to make sense of all this. At one point I was literally going to ditch my whole career to live in Buzios, a small Brazilian fishing village cum bohemian-chic resort on the Atlantic coast.

Fortunately, my Brazilian boyfriend at the time, Paulo, told me I was crazy and talked some sense into me. "Yeah, it's true, you are affected by your father's loss, but those traits and habits are now part of you and you have to 'own' that fact. You're responsible for curbing the beast that messes your life up."

After being a less than perfect parent myself, I was eventually able to understand that my father had done the best he could. Looking back at my own parenting efforts didn't conjure up a sense of pride. I had a lot of regrets to rectify and fences to mend. I've been through a helluva cleanup in recent years. It was like sweeping through the wreckage of a tsunami.

When I started my film career, I was taking on way too much. I really did have my hands full as an inexperienced young mother. Eventually I realized that it was pretty damn tough on my children, too. I don't regret striking out on my own all those years ago, but being away from home so often definitely took its toll on my kids. It certainly wasn't all a bed of roses for them. I know, because they've told me so.

My children and I have had some long, tear-soaked sessions. There was a lot of troubled water, if you know what I mean. It has to flow somewhere or you'll drown in it. There were moments when I've apologized for my shortcomings and begged for forgiveness. Sometimes I felt that a confession of guilt was righteously called for; and it encouraged them to open up to me.

During these discussions, I've hung in there and listened and listened and listened. Fortunately, it has led us to forge a deeper bond, to be more present for each other, and more trusting. Sometimes it seems that my daughter and son waited so long for me to really "see" them, that they almost gave up hope that I ever would. I, too, had been waiting on my end, in order for the dust to clear so that I could find the pieces of me that were still under wraps. When I was finally ready to come knocking, they opened the door and let me in, thank the good Lord.

For Damon and Tahnee, it took a long time for some of the walls to come down. Indeed, I will never be able to reconstitute all that was lost or heal all the wounds. But I am able to hear what each of them has to say.

I don't know if you can relate to any of this, but from what I've gathered among my friends who are parents, it's not uncommon to feel guilt over past shortcomings and to struggle with the notion that anything bad that happens to your kids could have been avoided if only *you* had done things differently. Plus, once a daughter and son grow up and become adults, it's just harder to connect. Nevertheless, in this imperfect world, my kids have long been the focus of my thoughts and prayers. For me, our coming together has been a crucial reawakening.

I don't want to betray any confidences, but during a series of long talks between my children and me, I became a kind of punching bag for how much hurt they felt. It was part of the healing process. Fortunately, from a more mature point of view, I've come away from this knowing that realistically, under the circumstances, I gave them all that I was capable of giving. At nineteen, I wasn't really suited to be a mother. This meant that in our threesome there was no *real adult* present. Was I lacking? Yes. But my children have their own life now and are fulfilling their own destiny. I'm here, if they need me, and now the lines between us are clear and wide open. I will always see them through a mother's eyes and am grateful for the privilege of having another chance to make amends.

Fortunately, going back over old memories isn't always about guilt and recrimination. I've shared some priceless, one-of-a-kind moments with both of them.

On the other side of Eden, Tahnee and I have spent some amazing times together. Recently, I found some pictures of us clowning around and had copies made for her. I thought I remembered when and where the photos were taken. I was sure we'd been in Anguilla at the time. But Tahnee remembered that we were in Mexico on a *Playboy* photo shoot. And she was right. She recalled almost every single detail of that trip. Reliving those moments together and comparing our recollections impressed me with how important such times spent together had been for both of us. It was thirty years ago.

While I was raising my two children, there were times when it would have been undeniably better to have their father there to intervene as only a masculine presence can. I remember once using the threat of military school on my son Damon, when he was a teenager. His behavior was becoming impossible for me to handle. I told him that if he kept it up, he was going to end up in a military academy. His reaction was, "Don't try to be my father." Boy, did he hit the nail on the head!

I knew immediately that I couldn't take him on. I couldn't possibly play both mother and father roles. I could barely handle my side of things.

My inability to manage my teenage son led me to enroll him in a very reputable private boarding school in Ojai—not a military academy. Damon was a good kid, but deep down he was understandably angry that he didn't have his father around, and this was his rebellious period. When visiting my son in his dorm one day with the headmaster, I couldn't get through to him. It seemed that he was closing me out. My heart sank. The message was clear: "Don't even try it,

Mom. You can't do anything to control me now. I'm beyond that." He was seventeen.

Experiences like that have made me reevaluate my old-school father who kicked butt and put the fear of God into me. Painful as it was, in some ways, I was the recipient of the good side of his discipline. On occasion, it almost seems preferable to having your teenage son laugh in your face. I'd been hopelessly ineffective as a disciplinarian and usually backed off. I think the nannies were tougher on him than I was. But suddenly I was faced with a teenage son who needed an authority figure. Unfortunately, that person wasn't me. Katharine Hepburn once said that she never got married and had children because she was married to her career. I understand why. I doubt that there's a career woman alive who hasn't discovered that you cannot have it all.

Raising Kids on the Fly

It was vitally important that I travel abroad for my film career, which presented a whole new set of problems for our little family. When I began making movies, the nucleus of the film industry was in Europe. It wasn't in Hollywood anymore. From the mid-'60s through the early '70s it had moved to London, Paris, and Rome. New Wave cinema was taking the lead with films like *A Man and a Woman*, *Blow Up*, *Alfie*, and *Darling*. Most of the producers left in Hollywood were getting rather long in the tooth. The '60s youth explosion was shaping a new direction in filmmaking.

Obviously I had to be in Europe, and I didn't know how to arrange visitation rights for my children and their father across the continents. Often they went with me to these foreign countries. And too, I had been seriously involved with another man, who became a kind of surrogate father to my kids, though he was not the father they wanted. This complicated things even further, because I was the one who had custody of the kids.

One thing I'm sure of: the movie business is no place to raise children. Without a father, there was no one I could entrust them to who could possibly substitute for me as their parent. As a result, my children often saw me at the end of a seventeen-hour day when I was exhausted and dragging, or leaving for yet another location shoot for a long period away from home. For an almost three-year span, I worked six days a week filming and did photos every Sunday. During that time, a role reversal took place between me and my children. Whenever my kids found me feeling tired and blue, they unconsciously took on the role of parenting.

"It's gonna be all right, Mommy," they'd tell me. Then they'd entertain with one of their various routines for cheering me up. Tahnee used to rummage in my closet and come out wearing a hat, boa, and high heels and launch into one of her priceless numbers. Her favorite was the Helen Reddy song, "I am woman, hear me roar . . ." but she always got the words wrong. When it got to the chorus she sang: "I am strong, I am *invisible*. . ." It was so adorable, I could have eaten her up with a spoon. Those were the times when I would feel that being an actress was an awful choice. It wasn't compatible with real life at all.

Being on location then wasn't like it is today. I have read that now when an actress is pregnant or is a new mother during the course of a production, provisions are often made to accommodate her, such as a special trailer for a nursery, where she can visit her baby on her breaks. And filmmakers these days are sometimes willing to design a shooting schedule that works around a pregnancy. But back when I was raising my children, this could never have happened. There were no Brads and Angelinas adopting children and managing to be with them constantly, getting photographed with them and bringing them to the set. In my day, it was just not the accepted way of approaching movie making. Feminists or whoever is responsible for these innovations in favor of working actresses should be applauded. I say, bravo!

While I was unavailable on a set or on location, other people in my life started filling in for me not only with my children but with household decisions too. Once, for example, while I was away shooting a film, one of my husbands hired a decorator. When I came home, the entire house had been transformed. None of it had any connection to me whatsoever. What were these books, masquerading as antiques, doing on my shelves, anyway? It was like coming home to another film set. Or like that reality show, *Extreme Makeover: Architectural Digest Edition* . . . but instead of a needy family on the skids, the big surprise was unveiled for an overworked sex symbol who didn't have time to decorate. Ha!

Maybe the life I offered my children wasn't ideal. But it did have its upside. I hardly think you could equate my children to the abused characters in *Oliver Twist*, those orphans shunted from place to place. That wasn't really the case. There were reputable nannies and tutors who took care of them, and they were often taken on wonderful sightseeing trips that exposed them to architecture, to different cultures, to foreign languages, and to a level of sophistication uncommon for American kids their age. At one point, when I was doing British films, both my children attended Hampshire School in Knightsbridge. They came out of it referring to me as *Mummy*, in perfect little British accents! "Hello Mummy, may we have tuppence for chocolates?"

Obviously, my children grew up in a completely different environment than I had grown up in. I hadn't yet developed any mature parenting skills, whereas my mother was thirty years old when she had her first child, me. I did have a sense of responsibility, but my demeanor was more like an older sister's. I'd flip into authoritative mommy mode when I felt it was needed, but it usually caused a perplexed reaction; like *Huh?*

Because I was young and attractive and enjoying a lot of notoriety in my profession, I had to watch myself in order to avoid doing something inappropriate as their mother. Once I showed up dressed in a pair of tight jeans and thigh-high boots for a parent-teacher meeting on the campus of Tahnee's private school for girls in Bel Air, and it created a stir. Afterward all the girls at the school said, "Oh, Tahnee, your mom was here and you wouldn't believe what she was wearing! Hey, we saw that movie where she was kissing that guy. Did she really kiss him like that? Because it sure looked real." Tahnee, of course, didn't enjoy such remarks. I had to make a distinction between how I appeared in the role of Tahnee's mother and how I presented myself professionally.

There were men in my life who valiantly tried to shoulder some of the responsibility for my children. My second husband attempted to take on the role of father and assert his authority to some extent. He was reasonably successful for a couple of years, but he wasn't the same as their real father. I think that even very, very small children are surprisingly perceptive. My kids knew that the only reason he was with them was because of his desire to be with me. Meanwhile, their real father was hovering in the wings, which created even more ambivalence and confusion in their heads. And I was paralyzed, without a clue what to do.

The Aftermath of Divorce

I think some of you will agree that the repercussions of divorce sometimes seem endless. No matter how reassuring either parent tries to be, children are bound to suffer the worst trauma. I know this because I've experienced divorce from both ends, as the child of divorced parents and as a parent who got divorced. But in the case of my parents, I was already nearly grown up when my mother left my father. I even played a role in how it happened.

In describing my family life, I've painted my mother as somewhat passive and obedient to my father, at least until I intervened and told him to stop bullying her. Even so, this is an unbalanced picture. My mom may have given in to my father, but only to preserve our family. Inside, she never lost sight of her priorities. She was some iron butterfly! I myself thought she was paying too high a price to keep the family together. But now I understand the value of what she was doing—in spades.

Before my father, Mom had been deeply in love with a young man she met at college. They were even engaged to be married. When that romance broke up, she was devastated. That was when my father came into the picture and began wooing her.

When I reached the age of fifteen, my mother confided to me, as the eldest, that her marriage to my father was "on the rebound." She also revealed that she'd kept pictures of her first love, Bill, ferreted away in a secret drawer for all the years she'd been married. When she showed me these keepsakes, I began wondering why she stayed with my father. By this time all of us were very familiar with his bad temper. One day I blurted out the question, "Why in the world don't you take us and leave?" Mom's answer was, "Oh, no, I can't do that until you children are out of school." But more and more often, she would go to the drawer and get the secret packet out and show me the pictures of Bill and reminisce. "This is the man I was in love with, but his parents interfered."

During my senior year in high school, the most remarkable thing happened. I spotted a notice in the *La Jolla Light* newspaper announcing the marriage of a classmate of mine—a certain Judy Hoyt. Mom looked at the article and was astonished by what she read. "Oh, my God, it says here that her father is William P. Hoyt!" It was the name of her long-lost love whom she'd been engaged to in college. And he was living just a mile away from us in La Jolla!

I took the initiative to call Judy and find out if her father was the same William P. Hoyt who had gone to school with my mother. Judy didn't know, but she put her dad on the phone, and I signaled Mom to get on the line with him.

It was one of those moments when you could really believe in modern-day miracles. Not only was it the same Bill Hoyt, but as it turned out, he was separating from his wife, Virginia, for the second time and living at home just until Judy graduated. Then he was moving out.

It was during my senior year that my mother and William P. Hoyt began seeing each other again. By the time I graduated, she had left my father and filed for divorce. As she saw it, after close to twenty years, the Good Lord had relocated the love of her life and put him less than a mile away. She saw no reason not to take this as a good omen. The two of them were clearly meant to be together.

Fortunately, my siblings and I were grown up or almost grown when our parents split. I was seventeen. Even so, it disrupted our lives in a major way. My brother, who had borne the brunt of most of Dad's corporal punishment, was only fifteen. He was obviously disturbed by the whole divorce thing. He left the house and began staying most of the time at a friend's, a mile down the beach. My younger sister Gayle and I stayed at home and kept going to school. Gayle had had it. She was glad that Dad wasn't around anymore.

Even though my mother was now free of my father, she didn't get married right away. She wasn't that kind of person. There was a whole waiting period for the divorce to be final and a courtship period between Bill and her that needed to run its course. We didn't see a lot of him because Mom didn't bring him home. She never flaunted him in our faces.

Sometime after my graduation from high school, Mom finally married him. On the surface, my siblings and I adapted well to everything. But my mother's divorce did affect me strongly. Once I left home, I was absolutely determined to hold out for real romance. Whoever the man of my dreams was, our love for each other was going to be passionate. I wasn't going to make compromises like my mother had. In reality, of course, there is no perfect choice, no perfect couple, or perfect family. I'd have to endure the consequences of my own choices in men for many years to come.

His Kids, Not Yours

Enduring the fallout from your own divorce is one thing. But it's a whole other Pandora's box if the man you're involved with is divorced or in the midst of getting one. For one thing, he may have children from another marriage, and it's next to impossible to determine what your relationship with them is going to be like.

My last husband, Richie Palmer, had an eight-year-old son we called Little Richie. My first view of the little guy was when he peeked out shyly from behind one of his daddy's legs, holding onto the trouser for dear life. Richie was adorable and so well behaved. I didn't see any problems ahead. He lived with his mother in the Bronx, and we lived in L.A.

At first, it seemed as if Little Richie was very excited about meeting the "new woman" in his father's life. He was delighted to act as best man for Big Richie when we got married. About 350 invitations were sent out, and we were planning a fairly big wedding. A photographer and reporter from *People* magazine were there to cover the ceremony. A bunch of paparazzi were camped out across the street from my house, something which Little Richie did not fail to notice. He was wide-eyed and overwhelmed by all the brouhaha and publicity.

Little Richie probably enjoyed the affair, but instinctually, I didn't think it was good for him. He was smart as a whip and streetwise beyond his years, but he was still just a kid. Kids need to know that there's a stable place where they fit in and belong. Someplace familiar that looks, feels, and smells like home—an identity they know they can count on. Little Richie's safe place had just gone all topsy-turvy, and he was becoming overinvested in the razzle-dazzle.

When Little Richie returned to the Bronx, he phoned his dad to announce that he was "ready to be a star." Clearly, he was growing into a real pistol. Then *that* issue of *People* magazine came out, and he riffled through the pages, hoping to see photos of himself. He was terribly disappointed to discover that he didn't appear in even one shot!

Nonetheless, he had no intention of taking this lying down. So he telephoned *People* magazine and demanded to speak to the editor in chief, no less. When the guy came on the line, Little Richie asked him point-blank, "Where's my picture?" He couldn't understand why he wasn't included. "Who are all these people in the photos, anyway?" he wanted to know. "They aren't part of the family. I don't even recognize any of them. My father is the one getting married and I am the best man. I'm his son, too! So what's up?" We were all blown away. And, in a way, Little Richie was right. What moxie!

Richie's mom, Donna, was a lovely young woman who had raised her son to be well mannered. He was an excellent student in school and was loved by all his teachers. But after his mom remarried and had two more babies with her new husband, Little Richie was suddenly no longer the "one and only." That changed everything. With his strong personality, his episodes of acting out became much more frequent, and his mother was constantly on the phone asking Big Richie to step in.

When Little Richie came to visit us, it was a bit awkward for me, because I had very little authority over him. My only official parental role was that of "stepmother." All this was aggravated by the fact that he lived somewhere else, out of state. Most of the time, my husband was forced to administer long-distance fatherhood and secondhand discipline, which can lead to inconsistencies.

When the little guy became a teenager and could come to visit for longer, he'd look at me like I should go "get stuffed." I could see that he was conflicted, and he was always testing me. After all, it was his father he'd come to see; I was just the annoying third wheel. There were several moments when we ended up at odds.

The most memorable was the elevator incident. We had an elevator in our home, and when Little Richie was there, he liked to get into it and ride it up and down relentlessly. Potentially it was a dangerous thing to do. Who knew what could happen, if he pushed the wrong button? What if he got stuck between floors? We only used it occasionally, mainly for my luggage. But my stepson wanted to use it as a toy. Since Little Richie paid me no mind, the only option was to turn it off and take possession of the key.

He didn't like this strategy one bit, so he went to his father and demanded that it be turned back on. This was only one of many ways he challenged my authority, every step of the way. The saddest thing was that I knew what he was going through was a result of both his parents remarrying. But I was helpless to do anything about it. He even accused me of not liking him. It was probably the other way around.

My children were no different from Richie as soon as I began to date other men. I remember Tahnee going to the door one time and opening it to James Aubrey, the head of MGM studios, whom I was going out with. He was a tall, distinguished-looking gentleman. Tahnee gave him the once-over and blurted out, "Who the heck are you?"

"I'm Jim Aubrey," he answered, "and I've come to see your mother." Tahnee didn't back down a smidgen. "Let's get one thing straight," she said. "When you come to pick up Raquel Welch, you're picking up my mother." She was making it clear that she was not very happy about sharing me with somebody who was not her father. He was an outsider.

Maybe if Little Richie and I had had more opportunities to be together before he hit his teens, we might have found some common ground, or a bond between us might have formed. Eventually, his father would have tired of accommodating all his requests. I believe he did so because no father has the heart to come down hard with discipline when he doesn't see his son very often. In some situations, it probably is possible to change a child's perspective and win his respect over time. Maybe you really can become the adored stepmother. But the whole setup is a challenge.

An ever-rising divorce rate has certainly caused children a lot of pain and suffering. Getting married in the first place implies having kids and establishing a permanent home with bonds that hold a family together. In a fully committed arrangement, the parents don't disappear out of the picture, breaking up the basic family dynamic. Back in the day of the "good mother," few women had four husbands and boyfriends in between. Few men had different women coming and going. In my view, too many of us have fallen way short of that standard.

The Empty-Nest Syndrome

Whether you've gone through divorce or not, if you have children, you're bound to face an empty nest someday. It's inevitable that you'll find yourself wondering why they don't call more often. And when they do call, they don't really seem to tell you anything much, or answer your many questions. "Fine, Mother, I'm fine. I said, I'm fine, Mom, don't worry, I'm fine."

You may have done the same with your mother, but at this point, you may have begun to feel you're losing your connection with your children, which is a bit frightening, because they're really an extension of you. You're still overjoyed about anything they do and overly disappointed about every misstep that causes them to stumble. Even so, it's essential for you to find a whole different way of communicating with them. You've come to a stage in life where you have to develop that most difficult of all virtues: patience. And patience is usually accomplished with your mouth firmly closed.

At this stage of affairs, you should consider it natural that they're not going to divulge certain things to you. They'll imply them. It might be about something as important as a new relationship or a new job, or they have plans to move away and set up housekeeping out of state. Whether it's the East Coast or West Coast or London, you're gonna miss them. Nevertheless, you'll have to pick up clues from the way they behave with friends, or their particular energy level, or the expressions on their faces. We mothers can read signs that others can't see. The important thing is not to start feeling like the bystander, or the lowly spear-carrier in a gigantic opera company. You are not irrelevant. The fact that you're always available to listen still means more to them than you (or they) can express.

Be aware that you'll need to be the one to take the initiative if they don't call, but don't admonish them with "You said you'd call!" as if they're little kids. *All you have to do is be there.*

I discovered what a big deal just "being there" is when I finally lost my own mother. We tend to take our mothers for granted like the nose on our face. But when your nose is missing, boy, is there a void! You feel as if you can see right through into your own soul; and what you find is this huge need, this enormous loneliness, a kind of fear, a forecast of your own mortality.

At one point, I decided to make all my calls to my children joyful, and all my visits with them upbeat. I decided to stop being the worrying mother once and for all, because I knew it would worry them, too. They had even told me so: "Mom, I can't tell you things, 'cause I don't want you to worry."

Once I relinquished the worrying, I took great pleasure in just sitting across from my son and looking at him, thinking, "Oh God, he's the best, he's the greatest, he really is . . ." It's quite wonderful to sit and stare at a son and listen quietly to whatever he decides he wants to tell

you. (As long as I'm not prying, he tells me a lot.) When I don't inter-
rogate, it frees him. He tells me more! Recently my son called me, and
we stayed on the phone for a couple of hours, going over the ins and
outs of a problem he was having. At the end, I asked if there was anything he wanted to ask. He said, "No Mom, I just needed to talk." Trans-
lation: "I wanted you to listen." Of course, I don't always get it right.

Last April, I bought my daughter a crazy Easter card. While I was
addressing the card, my hand slipped, and I ended up writing "Tahnee
Welch," instead of just "Tahnee," like I usually do. When she picked up
the card, she noticed it immediately and said, "Why the last name?" And
I said that it had just happened that way, and I didn't want to start a
new envelope. Tahnee laughed and said, "I never told you this, Mom,
but all those years when I was a kid, sometimes you'd forget, and instead of signing, 'Mom,' you'd write 'Raquel,' and Damon and I used
to laugh about it. But it used to bother me."

When you sign lots and lots of autographs, you develop a slam-bam
way of writing your name, and you don't even think about it. But when
it came to my daughter, using her full name had obviously stirred up her
past suspicion that I didn't think of her as special. Of course this is all
conjecture, but it serves as a reminder that childhood hurts die hard.

Nevertheless, no matter *how* perfect any mother is, there's always
cause for alienation between her and her children at various stages in
their development. There'll be times when they distrust and scoff at *anything* you try to offer. Then there'll be other times when they accuse you
of not offering enough.

My daughter took up photography when she was very young. She
was fourteen when she began shooting photographic portraits of her
classmates, as well as aspects of nature. I remember her doing a series
of photographs of her legs and feet wearing my high heels. She shot them
in the bathroom against the tile walls, and I realized that unconsciously
she'd been influenced by Helmut Newton! He'd been to our house and
photographed me in the backyard, so she was familiar with him. She'd
also been around movie sets and special photographers like Terry
O'Neill most of her life, which led to her fascination with photography.

Eventually, Tahnee began working on large collages. Using fragments of photographs, she created some surreal effects with dozens of eyes and lips floating throughout the frame. When I hung her artwork on the walls, she was nonplussed. "Oh, Mother!" she chided me. But I could see she was genuinely talented and definitely had an artistic eye.

When she was a few years older, someone who knew us both told me, "Tahnee is working with an acting coach and is going to an actors workshop, she's there all the time."

"She is?" I asked. She had never told me that she wanted to be an actress. Aren't mothers always the last to know? She did study diligently to be an actress, on her own terms and not as my daughter, and she became a really very fine one.

That's What Friends Are For

Maybe you feel this chapter has painted a rather dim view of a woman's social world, with all its talk of divorce and alienated children. I haven't intended to cast it in such a dark light. In fact, in my current stage of life, I've developed a taste for the richness of all kinds of friendships, many of which are outside of love relationships and outside the family circle.

During every period in my life, my girlfriends have played an important role. Their importance seems to increase as I get older and probably will for you, too, especially if you feel you're at a place in life when you're either in between partners or not interested in another relationship with a man. In such cases, it's likely your girlfriends will be the people you laugh with, share your disappointments with, shop with, and get another opinion from. They may also be the people responsible for broadening your horizons. I am always ready to hear about the wide range of experiences my friends are involved with.

Recently a friend of mine called to say she'd won $62,000 in a poker tournament and couldn't wait to tell us. Another friend I have is a writer. When she talks about her experiences, it opens up completely new worlds for me. She's extremely articulate, and in her own meticulous way knows more about the movie business than I do, because I don't keep as well informed about indie films as she does.

Looking back over the years, I realize that almost every single time I've hit a big snag with my husband or some significant other, a girlfriend has been there to help me sort through the wreckage. I could have talked to my mother about it, as well, but some things you tell your girlfriends, and other things you tell your mother. That's the way it is.

I admit that when I'm involved with a man, my girlfriends often get pushed to the back burner and I tend to adopt the man's circle of friends. This is something that still happens to most women. Quite often, a woman will socialize more with her husband's friends, if *he* prefers to gather with his own crowd. But it's a mistake to allow that to take over completely. I will never again neglect my close friends.

Other long-standing companions I value are my gay friends. They are some of my oldest and dearest relationships. But to be honest, I don't usually speak of either lesbians or gay men as a separate "group," because that's not how I see them.

There are a lot of straight guys who are not interested in certain kinds of things that I like. For example, I've found it next to impossible to drag a straight American man to a foreign film or to the ballet. But I have gay boyfriends who love to go and can thoroughly appreciate those experiences with me. In fact, when I was married and living in New York, I had a very close friend named Billy Barnes who used to go with me to lots of gallery openings and theater and was so much fun.

He was Tennessee Williams' agent and very knowledgeable about many subjects. He was also well traveled and extremely cultured. Billy was always fabulously turned out and very chic, a twinkling star on the New York social scene who was full of enthusiasm and had a sparkling wit.

Billy threw wonderful parties on his fabulous East Side roof garden. I met Arthur Miller there, and it was normal to run into Halston, Elsa Peretti, Ali MacGraw, Tennessee, Faye Dunaway, Al Pacino, or Bob Fosse. In fact, you could bump into almost anybody who was anybody there, from fashion glitterati to literary mavericks and movie stars. Unfortunately, Billy became an early casualty of AIDS. Such a heartbreaker. I will always remember him fondly.

A Fourth Chapter

I believe that in many ways we're lucky to be living in these times. In the past, the scope of a woman's life was predetermined to a large degree and divided into three chapters: girlhood, marriage, and motherhood. All three were quite narrowly defined. When these roles were over, life could seem sterile, and a woman might feel as if she were cast adrift. Now the possibilities are endless. You can get involved in just about anything that interests you. You can even go back to school and get a degree in an area that can lead to a later-life career.

As a new breed of older women, we're almost like pioneers, scouting out a new frontier, the span of which may consist of thirty years of leisure time. A fourth chapter has been added to our time on this earth to live, love, and learn. I say let's use it. Personally, I don't think I will ever retire 100 percent. I will always be busy doing something, keeping my hand in. Life is more interesting that way.

You'll notice that, as you grow older, there's a need to restructure your time, and new goals to fulfill. Maybe you always liked gardening, but you never really got the chance to do the kind of planting you wanted. Perhaps you've always wanted a vegetable garden. Well, now you can begin to plant those seeds. Who knows? If you're good at it, you could become a landscape designer.

You might be surprised to discover simple predilections that you never had the time to notice in yourself. Maybe you'll find out that you're a walker, or a writer, now that you have the time to do it. Maybe you'll like to express yourself as an artist, by painting with oils or watercolors. Maybe even though you always thought of yourself as unathletic, because you hated going to the gym, you might suddenly discover how much you like the fresh air and vigorous rhythm of a long hike. You'll begin to explore new canyons on camping trips or hiking expeditions, or while biking.

Greta Garbo loved to walk later in life and spent a regular portion of her days climbing through the Hollywood Hills. When she got to New York, she continued, walking through the streets in the early morning hours before they were crowded with people. She seemed to have a very limited interest in being part of the social scene. I can't say I blame her. She was a Virgo, and so am I. We're not afraid of solitude. When I read her autobiography, I found myself relating to her famous statement, "I *vant* to be alone."

I'm not drawn to a lot of socializing. I like more intimate groups of people, where I can really engage in conversation or take the time to get acquainted with someone new. But when it gets too massive, it becomes impersonal. A couple of black-tie, red-carpet events for charitable causes each year are enough for me. The Children's Diabetes Foundation's Carousel Ball, hosted by the adored Barbara Davis, is always great fun. The annual Met Gala in New York is fabulous, as is the annual *Vanity Fair* Oscar party, which is not to be missed. But unless you would be breaking a commitment, or missing something that is a professional obligation, what's the point in forcing yourself to become a social butterfly when it's really not your cup of tea?

A note of caution: Later in life, you're going to need to ask yourself, *What do I really like to do?* And if the answer is *nothing,* you're in big trouble. In fact, I doubt that's really the case. It doesn't have to be something you think you should be interested in, because now there's nobody to tell you what you should do, or what's socially acceptable. Find out what you really like and how you enjoy spending your time.

Take my brother as an example. He just left for Buenos Aires, because he loves the tango. For years he has been attending tango *milongas* (dance get-togethers) all over Southern California. The one in Buenos Aires is the most prestigious, where all the best dancers go. He is hooked on this style of dancing, and he likes the kind of international set that gravitates to the tango. When I finish this book, I think I'd like to take up ballroom dancing as well. It's a great way to stay fit. And I get a kick out of it. It's also a great way to meet people.

If dancing isn't your thing, animals may be. I know many people who are involved with animals in various ways. My sister belongs to a dog club for owners of the Cavalier King Charles spaniel, and she has forged many close friendships among them. Of course, there are always various traditional kinds of female activity, such as charities, or work with battered women and children. There are also museums and art gallery showings in every city and even memberships in those organizations.

Participating in projects that protect architectural landmarks can be a service to your community and, at the same time, an education in history and art. I was involved with the Los Angeles Conservancy, which attracts a number of people from the entertainment community, including Diane Keaton and Steve Martin. There was a drive to save certain landmark buildings that had been earmarked for demolition. Among them, the city of Los Angeles had made plans to tear down the legendary Ambassador Hotel. I had attended parties at the Coconut Grove, the famous celebrity showroom at that hotel, where stars like Bing Crosby, Frank Sinatra, Judy Garland, and Nat King Cole performed in their heyday. I'll never forget seeing Diahann Carroll perform there in the slinkiest of gowns, surrounded by palm trees. This was also the site where six early Academy Awards ceremonies were held, including the year *Gone with the Wind* and Vivien Leigh swept the Oscars. How could they even consider tearing this piece of history down?

Such thoughts were all the motivation I needed to get involved with the Conservancy, although they demolished that magnificent building, anyway. They tore it down and bulldozed it under. That's one West Coast trend I hate. The great cities of Europe protect and restore their famous edifices. When will Hollywood ever realize, before it's too late, that *the past is part of the present*? We are standing on the shoulders of those who came before. There are similar preservation groups in New York, and I suspect they exist in every major city. My grandfather was a prominent architect in Chicago, one of America's most beautiful cities, so I'm always sensitive to important architecture, whether from the Bauhaus, the Greco-Roman, or the Art Deco period.

Staying in Touch

Many moons ago, in the early '90s, my son said, "Mom, if you don't climb aboard the computer age, you are going to be left behind." My knee-jerk response was, "I don't want to know about it!" But of course, I did. So I started with baby steps almost twenty years ago. Now, of course, I'm at my computer all the time and constantly use it for research or to book theater tickets or plan the details of travel and vacations. I also visit YouTube, shop online, e-mail friends and conduct daily business through the Internet.

The trick is staying aware that there's a huge world out there. If you're a kid, you'll be compelled to master it. But when you're an adult, nobody is going to stop you from "checking out" from the rest of the world. I'm not talking about desperately trying to be younger and forcing yourself to use Twitter, join Facebook or try Internet dating. But aren't you curious? I'm referring to going where life leads you and having fun with it. It may be annoying, or even confusing at first, but if you don't stay mentally alert, you'll lose the ability to think straight. Think of your brain in the Nike sense. Use it or lose it. It's exhilarating when you discover what you're capable of accessing on the Internet. There's a fascinating new world out there waiting. Tap into it.

Here's something else to consider: just because you don't have children doesn't mean you could lose contact entirely with the next generation. What about your friends' children, for whom you can easily become an honorary auntie or godparent? It doesn't really matter how young or old you are. I have a girlfriend who has a darling son named Benjamin, and we keep up our relationship partly based on his birthdays and seasonal holidays, because Lisa's world revolves around being his mother. It's fun for me to hear news about him and go to his birthday parties. It fulfills the grandmother void in me. In fact, if you have the time, there are holiday festivities for very young children that you can get involved in all year long. Have you noticed that a lot of what's out there has to do with focusing on *others*? How great is that? It's often rewarding to take your gaze off yourself and direct it toward what you can offer to someone else.

For some of us, nothing beats travel. My sister is one of those vagabond travelers who can just pick up and go and is constantly enlivened by exotic places. She brings back paintings, hand crafts, videos, the whole works. She has a wonderful variety of amazing photographs showing the people and customs of Africa and Mexico. For Gayle, travel has become an edge-of-your-seat learning experience. She's passionate about her cultural field trips, and her enthusiasm for them is infectious. She's much more adventurous than I am when it comes to travel. I prefer some zen-like destination where I can lie on the beach and read—with my hat and sunscreen on, of course.

I may have cautioned you about not being intrusive when it comes to your grown-up children's affairs. But that doesn't mean it's out of bounds to travel with them and their partners, if they are up for it. One of my most enjoyable vacations was spent in Jamaica with my boyfriend at the time and my son and his wife. My son and daughter-in-law went their way, and we went ours. Then the four of us would meet up for Scrabble and later for dinner, but it was not compulsory. We all had a great time.

On occasion, my sister and I have gone to various places in Mexico and the Turks and Caicos islands, or to the British Grenadine islands. Since both of us are physical fitness buffs, we like to get up at the crack of dawn and go for endless walks or bicycle rides, before eating a healthy breakfast. In fact, the more you step away from the things that usually involve you in life and take a second look, the more ideas for simple pleasures spring to mind. This is such a huge country. There's nothing to stop you from getting into your car and just driving. From my home in Southern California, I can drive to Sedona, Arizona, or locations in Utah. Or I can simply drive up the coast into wine country. It's a blast.

Even though the possibilities are endless, I do have a couple of caveats. Stay clear of solitary activities when you first find yourself alone. They can lead to a scenario of perpetual isolation. Life is a progression. At each stage of it, you should *willfully decide how you're going to participate*. There's nothing worse than dropping out of sight and taking a downhill spiral, just because things have gotten ahead of you. The trick is always to step up to the plate and stay involved. Accept the challenge.

FOURTEEN

Mama Duck . . . Passing the Torch

LOOKING AHEAD AS EACH DAY PASSES, AND that spiteful clock keeps ticking, I don't want to miss this opportunity to pass along what I've learned to the next generation of young women. I've adopted a new role, which I call the Mama Duck syndrome—triggered by the fact that my own daughter doesn't listen to a thing I say. Will daughters ever learn? Will mothers ever tire of preaching to a deaf ear? But undeterred, I'd still like to pass along my perspective on what has happened to femininity, one that is seldom heard these days. So often over the past thirty years, I've looked in wonder at how the sexuality of women has changed. At one point I came to the conclusion that I didn't have good enough answers for why those changes had occurred. I began to examine the question from a broader perspective to understand how current sexual behavior evolved through the different waves of feminism from the suffragette movement on.

Women of my generation played a huge part in the '60s feminist revolution, but we were also shaped by the feminism that preceded us. Younger women may not recognize this, but feminist history has had a profound effect on their lives, just as it has on mine.

A Legacy of Resentment

History is rife with examples of how women have been oppressed, but I believe that we have needlessly carried the resentment of that past oppression into the present day. Our standing has changed so radically, I feel we should be able to take some pleasure in our newly exalted status and be thankful and humbled by the privileges we now enjoy. And yet for some, it would seem our accomplishments will never be enough to quell the anger.

I believe that there are certain fundamental biological and spiritual truths prescribed by the way male and female beings were created. I know that this view goes against the grain of most of what is being taught to young women in the halls of academia, where a *reformed idea of womanhood* is being absorbed by coeds who are looking for answers. In college courses about women and feminism, sometimes referred to as "womyn's studies," the current feminist philosophy comes through loud and clear; even in the spelling of *womyn*, which eradicates the single letter that connects women to men. In my view, at the heart of this mind-set is the notion that *men are the problem*. As someone who was resentful of my father's behavior, I certainly can sympathize with that sentiment, but only to a point; I refuse to blame my state of being on someone else. I have learned that finding fault elsewhere only serves to get you off the hook in your own mind, but eventually it renders you powerless to change your condition.

Let's examine this animosity toward men on its merits. Do centuries' worth of resentment women have held against men for ill treatment have any legitimacy? I think they do. I'm no scholar, but it's clear that as far back as ancient Greece and Rome, the dominant members of society (men) viewed women as chattel. Although they acknowledged the universal force of feminine power in the mythological goddesses Aphrodite/Venus, Athena, and Diana, and revered the feminine as an essential element of the cosmos, when it came down to the daily grind, they chose to suppress the female force in the human race, for fear it would rival male supremacy.

For many centuries, a woman's importance and standing rested to a large degree on that of her husband or father or on the protection she could secure from some patriarchal figure she might find favor with, usually on the basis of her sexual desirability. These days we call it "marrying well."

It took centuries for women to emerge from relative obscurity and finally realize their full potential. But eventually during the Middle Ages and the Renaissance women began to assume more and more important roles, not only in managing the home, but also in the world of trade, and even in politics. It was a period in history when one of my favorite heroines, Queen Elizabeth of England, came to prominence. On the world stage, she proved to be a formidable sovereign, commanding armies and ruling over men. Even as a young girl I was inspired by the idea of Queen Elizabeth facing off with the Spanish Armada, as Commander in Chief of the British Navy, when they annihilated the enemy fleet that threatened to invade their shores. I count her as a true female icon along with Jeanne d'Arc. It's no wonder that she has been portrayed so vividly by some of our most accomplished and colorful actresses, including Bette Davis, Helen Mirren, and Cate Blanchett. During Elizabeth's reign, it became easier for women to own property, to divorce, and to engage in business. Such trends carried over to the New World and eventually helped to establish a more level playing field for American women.

I don't mean to get bogged down in ancient history, but it's only in the light of the past that we learn to see ourselves objectively. Throughout history, women have been prey to exploitation and cruelty and were limited, with few exceptions, to the very small sphere of domestic activity. Nonetheless, by the twentieth century, we had cleverly maneuvered ourselves into positions of power.

We may still have a way to go, however; not just in terms of policy, law, and paychecks, but in our own hearts and minds. I believe the ghosts of our ancient oppression continue to haunt the current outlook held by women today, including hard-line feminists. Old wounds die hard and tend to dampen enthusiasm for all the positive changes that feminism has won for us. Women are a powerful force, and since much of that power has been unleashed in the Western world over the course of this past century, it's about time we gave some serious thought to where this force is taking us. It's time to stop whining and count our victories as blessings, without adopting the arrogance and sense of entitlement that were once identified with macho men. Nor should we hold on to a vision of ourselves as victims. Our demons lurk in the war of ideas inside our heads, and the cold war of the sexes still flares up and spills over into the home, the classroom, the boardroom, and not surprisingly, the bedroom, where some feisty women have adopted the role of sexual predator, so analogous to stereotypical male behavior.

"It's Sex O'Clock in America!"

The headline above sounds remarkably like something we might read today, doesn't it? But according to Carolyn McCulley, in her eye-opener of a book, *Radical Womanhood*, this provocative statement was emblazoned above an article in the *St. Louis Mirror* almost a century ago, in 1914! I can't help but compare this relic of a bygone era with the blatant and widespread worship of sex in American culture today. Though the new sexual openness of 1914 might look tame compared to what we're seeing now, *sex* seems to have become the official religion of the twenty-first century. Sex and money, money and sex, are the twin golden calves of our time.

Judging by our current lifestyles, doesn't it seem as if women today have come full circle and are returning to a time when the clock strikes sex again? Though women once held the moral reins and set the standards of acceptable behavior in the home and in society at large, we have now all but abandoned that role. In an earlier day, women went to church in search of higher meaning and moral guidance. But this kind of conscience and motivation to defend the greater good is no longer seen as a woman's particular province. Other priorities have captured our collective imagination.

Following on the heels of the suffragette movement and just two years after the provocative "Sex O'Clock" headline appeared, the controversial birth control advocate Margaret Sanger opened the first American family-planning clinic in the Brownsville neighborhood of Brooklyn, in 1916. And nothing would be the same again. Since that time the growing proliferation of birth control methods has had a profound effect on the sexual identity of women. Early in the century, Ms. Sanger had been vigorously campaigning for research into contraceptives and birth control, in any and all forms. She was inspired by the death of her own mother, who died while giving birth to her—the last of nine children. Not surprisingly, it was Sanger's opinion that her mother, an Irish Catholic, had been treated as little more than a baby-making machine, which contributed to her death by tuberculosis. Sanger's influence on birth control for women, in preventing unwanted-pregnancy and self-induced abortions, still endure long after her death in 1966.

Although Sanger was well intentioned, there were other implications that arose from her platform. To this day, concerns over tampering with the conception of a human life and qualms about abortion have had far-reaching consequences for both sexes and for society as a whole. Noble as family planning may be, the relentless push for more convenient and effective methods of contraception has led to a sea change in female moral values. One significant effect of the Pill on female sexual behavior was, and still is: "Now we can have sex anytime we want to, without the consequences. Hallelujah, let's party!"

By the early '60s, the dial-a-pack form of the Pill was on the open market. Some have argued that this innovation paved the way for the second great wave of feminism that followed in the 1960s. The one transformative power the Pill did have was to make it easier for a woman to delay having children until after she established herself in a career.

Nonetheless, for young women of childbearing age, there was a need for some careful soul-searching before addressing this very personal decision. A decision I too would have to face.

When I discovered I was pregnant at age nineteen, I panicked! Even though I was married to the baby's father, every fiber of my being went into shock. I wasn't ready for this. At the same time, since it was Jim's baby too, "the decision" was not mine alone to make. I had always wanted to have his babies, but not so soon. Talk about being in over my head. I'd been a fertile young virgin, and frankly, neither of us was very sophisticated about sex. I wasn't even sure we were doing it right . . . and *bam*, I got pregnant. When I realized that the cause of my nausea was not the flu, the mere thought of actually *giving birth* terrified me. That reality had never been part of my romantic fantasy. Still, I wasn't at all sure how Jim would react when I told him. Remember, we were both nineteen-year-old newlyweds, struggling to make ends meet. But he was unflinching in his desire to keep our baby and his positive, upbeat attitude about being a dad turned everything around! I have always loved Jim for how he responded in that moment. All that was left for me to deal with were my understandable qualms about having a huge big belly and the fear of excruciating pain of childbirth. It was a mega-adjustment to wrap my head around. The enormity of the entire ordeal, and the grave responsibility I'd be facing by having a baby, were overwhelming. Little did I anticipate that not too far down the road, I would be the mother of not one, but *two* children!

Teenagers constantly hear, "You have the world by the tail!" Before this happened, I wasn't yet cured of the arrogance of youth; now, for the first time, I was brought down to earth. I began to realize how helpless and foolish I must look in the eyes of God. Bearing a child seemed to affect every cell in my mind and body. The weird part is that the whole process *was not about me*. It was about the embryo and womb going through a metamorphosis so another life could be born. I was just a spectator. It came down to an act of self-sacrifice especially for me, as a woman. But both parents are fully involved, not just for that moment, but for the rest of their lives. And it's scary. You may think you can skirt around the issue and dodge the decision, but I've never known anyone who could. In our case, the decision to have a child was the best choice *we* could have made, and the sacred gift of our son and daughter has been an endless blessing to both of us.

The Second Wave

Just as I arrived in Hollywood, the *second wave* of twentieth-century feminism exploded. In 1963, the publication of Betty Friedan's book *The Feminine Mystique* became a pivotal part of the new women's movement. Her philosophy pitched "libbers" out of the confines of the home and motherhood and into the pursuit of a different kind of identity. By the '70s and '80s, a young woman's self-esteem and social standing would now rest primarily on her material and financial wealth and professional standing *outside the home*. But Friedan's message took a while to catch on, incongruous as it was to the new direction '60s pop culture was heading in.

"The times, they are a'changin'," predicted Bob Dylan, and indeed they were. In a few short years the widespread use of new birth control methods eventually mushroomed into a hedonistic surge of fearless sexual encounters, further fueled by pot, hallucinogens, coke, and heroin. I was living in London at the moment when the '60s generation erupted into a ribald revolution, kicked off by the Beatles, and later joined by Led Zeppelin, the Who, Jimi Hendrix, the Rolling Stones and others who expanded our consciousness with their music. And yet, while residing in Swingin' London, my monogamous instincts often ran in direct conflict to the wild lifestyles surrounding me. Although I was part of the scene, I was mainly drawn to the fabulous music and fashions. I stayed well clear of any drug use. Getting high with people I hardly knew was not for me. Besides, I didn't have time for shenanigans; I was working. Across the Channel in Paris and all over the U.S.A., there were political demonstrations and antiwar rallies; Martin Luther King Jr. was arrested for marching to abolish segregation in schools amid the shocking racism in the South. Much of what I thought I knew about my country was turned on its ear. It was a tumultuous and troubling time to be alive. Yet in spite of the chaotic events, which shook the world, I felt fortunate to experience this important period in history.

The '60s had an enormous effect on my personal life, my identity as an actress, and the way the public saw me. By 1966, I had a successful and demanding career, but it was not without the nagging guilt I carried daily over leaving my young children in the care of others. As I've said, in those days there weren't toddler-friendly nurseries and Mommy-breaks on movie sets. Dealing with '60s feminism *and* the onslaught of the sexual revolution wasn't always easy. The female side of my nature was in extreme conflict.

The irony is that though behind the scenes I was struggling to reconcile my career with my maternal obligations, my public persona was taking on a life of its own. My star surfaced on the horizon and I became an instant international sex symbol. Public reaction to my image on film and in photographs was off the hook. Everything about me was a definite departure from Marilyn's style and what had come before. I broke the mold of the soft blonde queen of the boudoir. I think the reason my image made such an impact is that I was an early *female* action heroine. Kind of like a female Clint Eastwood, without the cigar and six-shooter.

At this point, my sexy image was caught in a schism between the feminists and the hippies. They dubbed me "a sex symbol in the age of flower children." For an actress like me, with more moderate views, there was no place to land. In just a few more years, the whole essence of the "free love" doctrine would be epitomized by the 1969 Woodstock Music Festival, where thousands of naked young girls high on acid danced through muddy fields with their "wasted" partners in an orgy of abandon. They seemed to take Jim Morrison and the Doors literally, when they were called on to "break on through to the other side." Most of the hippie chicks thought it was groovy to be considered "sex objects." They were focused on loosening their sexual inhibitions, rather than on storming the halls of power. Simultaneously, feminist dogma continued to rail against male chauvinism and sexual exploitation, as well as the confines of marriage. The two-parent family was pushed to the back of the bus. Now there was nobody at home to mind the store, or to care for and raise the children. And that's where they lost me. For my part, a stable home for my kids became the top priority. To that end, I returned to L.A. from London in 1968 with my new husband, Patrick, who I hoped would provide my kids with a good father figure. My plan was to set up a suitable life for them in a more stable environment.

As early as 1969, the face of the women's lib movement was changing. A new feminist icon, known for her beauty as well as her intellect, appeared on the scene. She was Gloria Steinem, an aggressive journalist and publisher who was one of the editors of *New York* magazine. She had already broken feminist ground in 1963 with an anti-Hefner investigative report about how the women of *Playboy* were being exploited. She would go on to cofound *Ms.* magazine, one of the first mainstream publications to be devoted to feminist issues.

Gradually, with the influence of women like Steinem, the hippies and flower children of the '60s were transformed into the upwardly mobile, professional women of the mid-'70s and '80s. Women had also become physical culturists and, if necessary, could kick butt and take no prisoners. Contraceptives had by now become a way of life. Feminism was still going strong and was in no danger of stopping there, and I was changing, too.

I'd grown tired of the limits of strictly sex-symbol roles. So in 1969 I took a giant leap of faith and consented to play the lead in an audacious movie called *Myra Breckirridge*, which became a landmark in gay culture. The script was based on Gore Vidal's famous book of the same name. It was a surreal comedy that forecast the role reversal of the sexes. Vidal's controversial premise was inspired by the notion that the average man could no longer cope with or compete with the new superwoman (which feminism had produced) and that men in general were losing their dominance. So, amid a slew of clever script references to Hollywood's famous leading ladies of the '30s and '40s, as the story goes, an imaginative film critic, Myron Breckinridge played by Rex Reed, transforms himself into a transsexual female icon, played by me!

Unquestionably, the movie had its flaws, but you could say that the sexual duality behind the character of Myra/Myron Breckinridge was definitely way ahead of its time. Everywhere you look today, there are examples of men and even women who are undergoing gender reassignment surgery. Gore Vidal's book was definitely a harbinger of what was to come.

By the mid-'70s and early '80s, the Me generation began to emerge under the distressing cloud of HIV-AIDS. This would forever change the sex lives of an entire generation. In reaction to the sadness and fear that plagued those early years of this deadly epidemic, people allowed themselves to get swept up in the pulsating beat of the disco era. Club life ruled, as did Warhol's superstar iconic imagery and the appeal of anonymous groupie sex. For the entire decade of the '80s, after my stint on Broadway in *Woman of the Year*, I chose to make my home in the Big Apple, where I watched helplessly as some of my dearest friends succumbed to AIDS. I still miss them all terribly, and hope one day there will be a cure for this dreaded disease.

I really feel for younger women who have had to live with the threat of AIDS and other STDs since puberty. They have never known anything different. I can only imagine how treacherous dating and trusting a sexual partner must be. I consider myself fortunate to have spent my prime during a period when HIV and other dreaded diseases had not yet become a fact of life . . . and death.

Post Feminism—Pro Pornography

Up until the 1990s, members of the feminist movement, though sexually liberal, had been nearly unanimous in their censure of pornography. Women stood shoulder to shoulder, globally united in opposition to the porn industry. The proliferation and accessibility of pornography was condemned as degrading to women. I find it odd that since that time, the opposite is true. Many postfeminists of the '90s, in defiance of their predecessors, have embraced the porn industry as a profitable enterprise, protected by freedom of expression. It wasn't long before more and more women were starting to cultivate their skills at pole dancing, inking their bodies with tattoos, and adorning themselves with multiple piercings. Nothing against those who have made those choices. I respect their right to do so. But one cannot ignore that such customs were once confined to the underbelly of society and are now being adopted throughout mainstream culture.

Many of my friends who are parents of teenagers sat in stunned silence several years ago when it came to light that oral sex had become a popular practice among adolescent girls in middle schools across the country. The thirteen-year-old daughter of one of my friends readily admitted to performing fellatio on several boys at school on a regular basis. "Aw come on, Mom. It's no big deal. Everyone is doing it," she said. Apparently, if it's not the *act of intercourse*, kids don't count it as sex. Can any sane woman fail to make a judgment call about that?

One has to ask where the female voices of conscience are hiding in the face of these troubling trends. Doesn't the next generation of children need and deserve our protection? At the very least, young girls need to be taught (or cautioned) about the dangers of hooking up.

Hooking Up

According to the journalist Laura Sessions Stepp, in her excellent investigative book *Unhooked*, young women in their late teens and twenties seem to be caught up in a new kind of promiscuity. Stepp has interviewed young coeds extensively on college campuses, and she's found it's quite common for them to feel compelled by peer pressure to be more sexually aggressive than ever before. In order to live up to expectations, young girls are engaging in multiple sexual encounters, which they refer to as "hooking up," that have no meaning. They always take the initiative, thereby establishing an abrupt and uncomfortable role reversal. In their interviews these girls admit that this empty sexual behavior doesn't fulfill them. It certainly doesn't express love, or lead to it. It doesn't even guarantee good sex. So then why indulge in such practices?

Ironically, younger women today are facing a dilemma very similar to one that was typically faced by men with "commitment phobia." In a way, I can sympathize with younger women when they think, "Hey, I have a profession and a life without a man, so do I really want to make a commitment to a partner, a home, and motherhood? Consequently, if by mutual consent, my temporary male partner(s) and I *use each other*—simply because it's too difficult to abstain from sex for long periods—where's the harm?"

I understand the temptation, except that the idea of having casual sex with different partners—even in my younger days—always seemed totally out of bounds to me. Some might say that I'm confusing sex with love and vice versa. But I've always believed that the two belong together and are interdependent on one another, unless you suppress your female instinct. I've always identified no-strings sex as a male impulse. The catch is, if hooking up simply serves as an impersonal *skin fix* for lusty young girls, then why does the clinical research show that their unguarded feminine conscience tugs at their emotions and causes them grief?

I concur with Laura Stepp when she writes, "A girl can tuck a Trojan into her purse on a Saturday night, but there is no such device to protect her heart." She goes on to say that current "female sexual assertiveness mirrors—and even stems—partly from what they're showing in classrooms and on the playing field." By 1980, the percentage of American women enrolled in college topped the percentage of American men for the first time—52 to 48 percent. By 1990 the gap had widened to 55 to 45 percent, plus more women than men were enrolling in graduate programs. Nicely done, girls!

In the practical sense, I cannot see how a young woman can ignore such accomplishments over the past thirty years—as well as the career opportunities they bring. It's easy to see how greater opportunity might affect young women in their relationships with men. For today's ambitious young careerist, who has been programmed from childhood to define power on her own terms and defend it at all costs, it's hard to admit to an emotional need that seems buried in a bygone era. For her, the *need for a relationship* with a man is now prejudged as "old hat," and considered a sign of weakness.

And so the conflict between love and career remains an ongoing dilemma, as it was for me in my time. The difference is that the culture of *hooking up* dictates that women refrain from showing emotional vulnerability to their partner(s). Once you're independent, it seems like breaking an unspoken code of ethics to open your heart. And yet, is this proud posturing just the flip side of the classic power struggle between the sexes? After all is said and done, even today when a man and woman are about to split up and go their separate ways, their primary concern still remains, "Will I be the heartbreaker or the heartbreakee?"

Yes, there will always be an element of risk. No relationship that is centered on winning and ego can survive. No matter what your leanings, the fact remains that everyone is figuratively a loser when it comes to love and matters of the heart. The incurable romantic in me sides with the notion that the only solution is to join forces and collaborate. Finally, I don't believe it's possible to avoid facing the challenges inherent in being a woman. There are endless questions, and no easy solutions. A woman's ideal purpose and place in the world as it relates to the opposite sex will forever change, while each of us searches for the answer.

Reluctant Sex Symbol

I'm keenly aware that not everyone will share my opinions. They may seem judgmental or even preachy. I won't deny that I am passionate about the role of women and younger readers may think, "What does she know? She grew up in an age with a completely different set of values." On the other hand, women closer to my age might ask themselves quite the opposite question: "What right does a sex symbol who appeared before millions of horny men in a skimpy bikini have to tell us about the cheapening effects of sex on today's morals?" Well, fair enough.

My answer to that would be, that it's *because* of my mistakes and my triumph over the odds that I've learned how sexuality can obscure other qualities in a person and can pull the purpose of one's life completely off course. In my teens, I was drawn to the world of ideas: philosophy, theology, metaphysics. Had I not become distracted from my natural leanings, things might have been different. But once the beauty card came into play, I became addicted to the attention and influence it brought. I began to rely on it because it opened so many doors to my chosen career. And to a degree, I got caught up in that world—sex appeal is an integral part of the entertainment business.

If you're a sensual person like me, there's a natural attraction to the world of beauty, but also an aversion to being treated as an object rather than a person. It's a fine line to walk. I love my profession and have struggled as an actress to win the respect of my peers and attract better roles. However, sometimes I turned down important parts that would have raised my status as an actress, because I was uncomfortable with the moral message of the film. I felt compelled to stay true to my personal sense of integrity, and was conscious of the fact that my actions set an example for my kids and others. The role of an artist is often nonjudgmental—like an empty vessel—in order to take on the qualities of any character and to follow direction. But it's also important for me to fully commit to the overriding *message* of the project.

I can't help but identify vicariously with the new crop of girls tiptoeing through the dangers of sudden fame, knowing what I do about the inevitable disappointment that comes when reality sets in. Once you catch the brass ring, there are endless compromises to make. Any idealism you start out with takes a slap in the face. I got caught up in an exploitative business, but I eventually made my peace with my image and made it work for me.

Because of my image, there was constant pressure on me to appear nude on camera. Believe me that it was a precarious position to be in. The usual ambush went something like: "Here's where you open your blouse and expose your breasts." Or: "In this scene, we'd, um, like you to come out of the shower and drop your towel." They would always add, "Don't worry. We want you to be comfortable. It'll be just the camera crew, and we'll only shoot you from an artistic angle. It will be extremely tasteful."

Maybe they thought I was stupid. But one thing was certain, whenever I refused to get naked or climb into bed nude with an actor, I was labeled "difficult." I could always sense when they were ready to make their move. First came the "trust me" talk with the director. Then the producer would come in; then a call came from my agent, who would pressure me. And then the head of the studio would be on the phone, insisting that nudity was "absolutely necessary" for the scene to work.

My answer was always the same. I didn't agree that nudity was called for. There were lots of ways we could handle the action that would leave more to the imagination. The principle I held to was the precedent set by all the great film actresses before me, none of whom had ever appeared nude or done explicit sex scenes. The movies I revere, from *Casablanca* to *Doctor Zhivago*, contain some of the most passionate moments on film, where "a kiss is still a kiss." And those scenes still elicit moans of longing from viewers, even in 2010. Women today still ask one another, "Is he a good kisser?" because the answer usually tells it all. So why go to such extremes?

Remember, most of my early experience in the film industry was in the '60s and '70s, when codes of decency were crumbling, though it wasn't exclusive to me. Personally, I always hated feeling so exposed and vulnerable. I knew that I was expected to be "sexy," but reminded myself that, as provocative as Marilyn Monroe was, she never once appeared nude in her movies. There was the *illusion* of nudity when she pushed the envelope with her sheer Orry-Kelly costumes in *Some Like It Hot*, and that illusion was enough. I steer clear of judging other actresses who have appeared nude. Some of them are extremely talented and I'm a fan of their work. But I object to nudity being a prerequisite for all actresses, a "standard" that was born during the '60s.

I will concede that I've often cooperated with what the industry required of me in the roles I've played. I've definitely used my body and sex appeal to advantage in my work, but always within limits. Certainly my looks were an essential building block of my career. However, I feel strongly that a woman's mystery is part of her appeal; and the power of the imagination is more potent and provocative than graphic on-camera sex or explicit nudity. I reserve some things for my private life, and they are not for sale. For me, it's an invasion of privacy.

The issue of how much exposure is enough came up several times for me during the filming in Spain of *100 Rifles* (1969), a western with Burt Reynolds and Jim Brown that had an interesting biracial romance between my character and Jim's. When Tommy Gries, the director, wanted me to strip down and run stark naked through the Spanish desert with a pump-action shotgun, I just couldn't picture myself doing it! It would have been a career move in the wrong direction, and I'd have to do things that were more and more outrageous the next time, and the next. I had to admit that it was a potent image, reminiscent of a Sam Peckinpah slow-motion shoot-'em-up movie. But this sort of daring, in my opinion, would be better enacted by a female character who wasn't the lead; because after a stunt like that, who would be able to look at the heroine—me—without a smirk? I tried to find another solution.

The scene was meant to begin with me stopping a moving train by taking a shower under a water tower. I argued that my character, who was traveling with a group of rough riders, wouldn't risk exposing herself so openly. It might incite a dangerous reaction that she'd be incapable of handling. I suggested that my character (a Mexican revolutionary) could be standing under the water tower just cooling off, and that she could keep her shirt on as the water poured down over her body. In the period between 1910 and 1920, when the Mexican Revolution took place, the suggestive outline of her figure through the wet shirt would surely have been enough to stop a train of Federale soldiers. Then I'd pick up the shotgun and blow my opponents away. Fortunately, I won the argument. They ended up shooting the scene that way.

Right before I started shooting *The Three Musketeers* (1973), in which I was given a rare chance to show my comedic talents, I was offered a script for another film in galley form, based on a book called *The Fan Club* by Irving Wallace, about the kidnapping and gang rape of a famous actress by demented fans. The agents and producers involved in the project were proud to boast that it would stretch the boundaries of sexual propriety more than any other movie to date. They felt certain that it would clean up at the box office.

After I read only a few pages of the galleys, I slammed them down and called my boyfriend, Ron Talsky, to confide my feelings. "I'm so insulted!" I complained. "How could they think I'd be interested in doing this piece of garbage?" I was repulsed by the whole concept and horrified by the kind of disregard they had for me. I put the script in a box and sent it back to my agent at the time, Guy McElwaine, with instructions to tell whoever had sent it to go to hell.

Well, you wouldn't believe the result.

As soon as I finished filming *Musketeers* in Spain, the *same* salacious script arrived *again*. This time it was delivered in person to my home by three or four agents from the company that represented me. They didn't mince words.

"Here's the thing. You *gotta* do this film," they informed me bluntly, "because we've gotten you the biggest payday for this movie that has ever been offered!" They were quoting several million in salary, which was outrageous for the time. No actress in the movie industry had ever received that large a fee. "It's gonna push you way over the top!" my visitors assured me. "You'll be the biggest female star ever."

"Really?" I shot back, trying to swallow my rage. "What about my reputation . . . and what am I supposed to tell my kids? Not to mention my parents? They'll never be able to live it down! I'll never be able to hold my head up again. I have no interest in your friggin' script, for any fee."

But they persisted! "Okay, here's the deal. You go through the script and mark the sex passages you don't want to do. We'll get a body double to do them for you." What a sick twist! No matter which way I turned, the situation stank. There was no way I wanted to be associated with that trash.

Their next strategy was to threaten to send it to Brigitte Bardot instead. "Please do," I encouraged them. She, of course, turned it down as well. Then, believe it or not, the same people sent the material to me a third time! This time their attitude was nastier. "Do you know what the life span of a sex symbol is in this business?" they bullied. "It's short. Very short. So you know, Raquel, you should cash in on your image before it's too late." (I was thirty-four.) "The producer is a very tasteful man and we've watered the thing way down. Now there are only six rape scenes instead of ten!"

Once again they refused to take no for an answer. I was told I was making a big mistake. Overnight, I moved into a whole new category: I was branded as "trouble." I didn't have their support anymore. But with friends like those, who needed enemies?

One might think that tons of actresses would jump at the chance to strip down for that kind of money, and in years since, many have. But I knew the reason the script kept resurfacing: nobody else wanted to touch it. I guess I wasn't the only "prude."

After I had starred successfully in several terrific films, including *The Three Musketeers* and its sequel, *The Last of Sheila,* and *Kansas City Bomber*, I thought I had finally rescued myself from the SSS (sex symbol stigma). But I had underestimated the staying power of that label. In 1975, I signed on to appear in the Merchant-Ivory film *The Wild Party*, based on a rather dark narrative poem written in the 1920s by Joseph Moncure March. It is the story of a Jazz Age party that culminates in a murder. The plot was based loosely on a real-life scandal linking the silent-film star Fatty Arbuckle to the obscene death of a starlet. The talented James Coco played the Arbuckle role.

Appearing in a prestigious Merchant-Ivory film was quite an opportunity, I thought, and I couldn't wait to get started. They were considered serious artists, and would later win an Oscar for *A Room with a View* in 1987. You can imagine my astonishment when we came to the last week of shooting and James Ivory demanded I remove all my clothes for a brief bedroom scene. For me, it was like a recurring nightmare. As Ivory saw it, the scene required me to appear in the nude; he said it was "reality" he was looking for, not some Hollywood version of it. However, it was obvious to me that it was just a throwaway scene that Ivory planned to "milk" by adding nudity.

European films often have a lot of natural sensuality to them, and nudity has been common in the mainstream media there for quite some time. However, I'm an American actress, and nudity is viewed very differently here. At the time of the shooting of *The Wild Party*, America was still the place where the commercial standards for film were set. Plus, this movie was being released under the banner of American International Films, which couldn't claim any "artsy" European credentials.

My back was to the wall once again, as Ivory insisted that the scene had been there in the original script. "It didn't say naked," I countered.

"What else would you be, if you had just made love to some guy in that bed?" he answered testily.

I was torn. I loved Ivory's work and knew that he had an artistic eye, so I didn't want to oppose him. A voice in my head prodded, "Shall I do it for the sake of art?" This was a hard one.

Next my agent called me to say that I was ruining my reputation by refusing, and that it was going to keep me from working. All I had left to say was that if my not being naked in this film was going to make it boring, then so be it. I knew very well that the movie had to stand on its own merits. So we shot the less-than-three-minute scene without nudity. A small victory; but no one can resist such pressure indefinitely, and I was beginning to feel like I had somehow brought the conflict on myself. Had I been encouraging this sex symbol image . . . and now wasn't delivering on the bargain? People don't realize how difficult it is to steer one's career clear of the mire and still stay afloat. In times like these, I wondered if I'd survive.

Luckily, the success of several of my films proved that I would. *The Three Musketeers* turned out to be that summer's blockbuster and confirmed to everyone, critics included, that I had more to give. It had a superb cast that included Faye Dunaway, Oliver Reed, Richard Chamberlain, Michael York, Spike Milligan, and Charlton Heston. When I first read the script, I wasn't convinced of the comedy merits of my role. I had to trip and fall down constantly, over and over again, in every scene, for no apparent reason. I didn't get it at first. Nor did I realize that Dick Lester, the creator and director of all this slapstick nonsense, was a bona fide genius and that he was about to tap into a comedic streak in me that I didn't even know I had.

The film opened to raves. I found myself sneaking into the back of a theater in Westwood just to confirm to myself that it was true that I was funny. When the audience howled, I had to pinch myself. My performance cracked everyone up, and I won a Golden Globe for best actress! But even the charming Dick Lester, whom everyone adored, had wanted me to stick my tits through a carriage window so that some royal twit riding inside the coach could tweak them. I refused, and he used a double. Better her than me, thank you very much. But I still love the guy. Always will.

Women's Voices—Women's Values

I'm far from a paragon of virtue, above reproach. Nor in my day did I set such an impeccable example. But I've consistently tried to send the message that women should carry themselves with pride and that they are not just ripe for the picking.

I also know that, in the sea of opinions glutting the Internet, my point of view is but a whisper. And I can already hear the cries of protest. *Who does she think she is? Is she suggesting that we don't need freedom of speech and expression?* Of course not. But I don't always see those freedoms exercised with reason and responsibility. They are often exploited so that they work against the very principles they were meant to protect.

Fortunately, there is a host of admired female stars who have embraced their fame with style and class and have held to their own standards: Jennifer Aniston, Charlize Theron, Beyoncé, Gwyneth Paltrow,

Cameron Diaz, and Reese Witherspoon spring to mind. I tip my hat to them for carrying themselves with poise and dignity. They've set a valuable example for millions of female fans. I've even noticed what I hope is a new trend: many young professional women have put a premium on family and parenthood. What a welcome relief.

Seriously, folks, if an aging sex symbol like me starts waving the red flag of caution over how low moral standards have plummeted, you know it's gotta be pretty bad. In fact, it's precisely because of the sexy image I've had that it's important for me to speak out and say, *Wake up and take a long hard look at what's going down.*

AFTERWORD

The Spiritual Woman

WRITING THIS BOOK HAS BEEN QUITE AN odyssey. As each chapter unfolded, I imagined that I was sharing a personal journey with you and we were careening along a sometimes unexpected road together. I've relived some of my memories on paper in an attempt to diagram the experience of being a woman as I know it. After all, we women can truly benefit from a compass and a map to guide us through the different crossroads of our lives, especially in those areas outside the realm of hair, makeup, and the usual "drag." I thank you for indulging me in those opinions where perhaps we don't see eye to eye. But pretending not to have a personal point of view about the roles of women today and how we've changed, especially when it's such a hot topic, is just not an option for me. I'm too feisty for that. In reflecting on the essence of feminity, from the material to the spiritual girl, I'm compelled to turn my gaze now to the future and what awaits me around the next corner.

Moving On

It's wonderfully revealing to be left to one's own devices, undistracted. It's an ongoing exercise in self-discovery! Now that I'm outside the prism of seeing myself in terms of career, men, and physical appearance, my newly found free time has uncovered a hidden trove of buried treasure. I recently sold my house—a Tuscan-like palazzo that was starting to remind me of that huge empty shell of a mansion in *Sunset Boulevard*. Only ten years ago, Hutton House had represented my dream of a forever home in which I could be endlessly happy. But gradually my dream home morphed into something akin to a mausoleum. The palazzo had taken on the air of an epitaphic ending. I was feeling far *too* safe inside the gated palace walls with closed-circuit security cameras . . . I realized that I don't always like what is "safe." Rattling around inside this monumental paean to black-'n'-white Hollywood glamour, I wondered why the Norma Desmond staircase and the twenty-five-foot ceilings didn't satisfy my longings.

Luckily, I sold Hutton House at the top of the housing market and am now in transition, looking around for the next place to land . . . but I'm in no hurry and have leased a house not far from the palazzo so that I don't feel displaced or need to learn any new driving routes. It was an ordeal to orchestrate everything. Moving can be traumatic, but it can also be cleansing. As I began unpacking box after box in my new digs, sifting through the endless cardboard tombs that held the ghosts of my past, it seemed like an endless task. It took time to collect and organize all the scattered pictures, clippings, keepsakes, and scrapbooks that made up the unfinished jigsaw of my life. With the clarity of distance, I could now see many of those captured moments from a clearer perspective. It was a strange feeling, going over the imprints of my former self. Sometimes I laughed out loud, and at other times I cried. There was a tendency to want to edit out all the mistakes, but it was quite something to relive how I felt back then and recognize how incredibly caught up in the heat of the moment I had been, unable to see the forest for the trees. I'm not *HER* anymore.

What occurred to me is how the intensity of public scrutiny had robbed me of the enjoyment I might have savored on my own. I was more frightened and strained than I should have been, unable to let go of the striving and yearning to prove myself worthy. I hadn't been "in the moment," to use an acting term; I was too busy judging myself, maybe too harshly. Close friends had always called me on that tendency. "Rocky, don't be so hard on yourself." Where's the fun in that? Now I'm free to enjoy those experiences more in retrospect. Perhaps it's true that youth is wasted on the young. Today I realize that I didn't appreciate what I had. I was often incapable of being thankful for all the gifts that were lavished on me, which proved to be a hindrance. It hardened my heart, made me suspicious of the handlers and "users," constantly wary of ulterior motives. Yes, dangers were lurking, and I wasn't paranoid or hallucinating; but I made the mistake of taking all of it too personally. Going forward, I've made a vow to really open my heart up to my innermost thoughts and to that same inner self in others. There is so much to love and to embrace in this world.

Will I ever really see myself objectively? Fat chance! Many do claim understanding as they grow older. Since the human condition so often breeds the same mistakes over and over again, I suppose we older types are bound to learn to avoid certain pitfalls. However, our kind of experienced wisdom is best conferred on others, who might benefit from our advice and whom we can see more clearly than we see ourselves. True wisdom, more often than not, is the sure acknowledgment that *we don't know . . . that we are not in control.* I'm reminded of the arrogance of my youth when I imagined I was the master of my own destiny. No wonder I got stopped cold more than a few times. A little humility opens the door to seeing things more clearly. It turns out that we cannot learn as much while imposing—or forcing—our personal *will* on circumstances. A revelation came with that discovery: the less I want for myself and the more I appreciate whatever I get, the more opportunities are forthcoming! It's as though we humans need to get out of our own way. And put ourselves in God's hands.

Searching for Answers

In the past ten years of my life, my direction has shifted significantly. I find that I'm less focused on the material and practical side of things and have begun to lean more toward finding spiritual answers, no longer content to drift. This has evolved in a very gradual way, through different stages of my life. I think it was inevitable because, like many of you, I've had to face the death and loss of loved ones, in particular my mother. With that moment came the contemplation of the hereafter. When my tears had dried over her passing, I couldn't stop thinking about what lies beyond that last breath. Strangely enough, I didn't find these thoughts morbid. Instead I found them welcoming and uplifting. I felt like a kid again, wanting desperately to know, *who* made the sky? What is God? And if he exists, I wondered what he had in mind for me. Questions and curiosity about the larger questions are not tolerated in adults and these days only indulged in children. And yet, throughout our lives, the answers remain elusive . . . or are we merely avoiding them?

Three years ago I found myself at the bedside of my beautiful sister, who had undergone surgery for ovarian cancer. As I gazed down at her sedated face, I began to pray: "Please dear God, don't take her away from me." I studied her familiar features and could feel her spirit everywhere in the room around me. At that moment, I was prepared to believe that there was something more than this lifetime . . . there had to be. Some things never die. It wasn't logic that brought me to this sense of infinity. I allowed myself to experience a primal instinct higher than thought. Call it a sense of wonder, that only a child would embrace.

I asked for a miracle. The surgery had taken seven long hours and she had been moved to the cardiology wing of the intensive care unit. I was worried by the grave expressions on the doctors' faces. But God was merciful. Three short years later, Gayle has made an amazing recovery and has no sign of ovarian cancer. In fact, she just came back from a trip to Croatia that most thirty-year-olds wouldn't undertake. I'm not saying this was a miracle, but I'm convinced that when people pray in earnest, believing, it does make a difference. And why not? Some forces are beyond our understanding. As Pascal once declared, "The heart has its reasons, which reason knows nothing of." What I do know is that Gayle will always be with me, in this world and the next . . . God willing.

On the day my mother died, some years ago, I felt as if I'd lost my only connection with God's favor. I figured that any standing I had in the hereafter was based on the life she led, not on my inadequate attempts at following His principles. At the same time, I was reminded of my own mortality. I also thought back to the countless times she had taken me to church as a child and remembered the wonderful sense of peace I'd felt when sitting under the protection and grace of my mother's faith. Now that I had lost my bearings, I wanted to reach out and touch the strong arm of God again.

It had been more than fifty years since I attended church. Up until then, a token twice-a-year obligation to sit in a pew for the holidays was enough to salve my conscience. But I didn't belong to any church now, and I was rather ashamed of myself. I managed an awkward inept prayer to ask where I should look for such a sanctuary. It was embarrassing. I wasn't sure exactly whom I was praying to anymore. So I prayed to the God of my childhood and, lo and behold, he was still there. My journey had just begun.

Then one Sunday morning, I drove down the freeway quite a distance outside of Beverly Hills. I found a beautiful little church on the way to Pasadena, where the pastor and congregation were very devout and really knew their scripture. I had come there because I'd heard the pastor speak on the radio, and it sounded like he might be a good source of information. That turned out to be true. Apparently, even inept, awkward prayers are answered.

The people in this church weren't Hollywood types. They were modest, unassuming, cheerful and friendly. They welcomed me. Even so, when I entered the chapel on that first day, I felt quite tentative. Maybe I didn't belong among these people who actually practiced their faith. I didn't look like them, sound like them, or act like them. I stood out like a sore thumb. So I took a seat in the back.

By the time the sermon was over, I felt remarkably comfortable sitting among these parishioners; not one of them gave me a second look. They were what my mother would call no-nonsense kind of people. Not a superficial bone in their body. How refreshing!

This is my church now. I have become a member of this parish and its people are my brothers and sisters in faith. Together we form a fellowship where I can reaffirm my beliefs and worship every Sunday. When I'm in their midst, I'm just Raquel, not anybody special.

If you take nothing else away from this book may it be a sense of new beginnings as you move forward in life. May you have the spirit to form your own opinions and the independence not to get swept along by the herd when your instincts tell you otherwise. Most of all, I sincerely hope that each one of you finds the answers to your most ardent questions. May those answers bring comfort to your heart and fulfill your soul.

The End

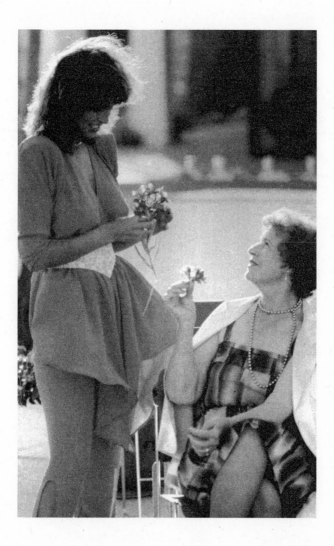

Acknowledgments

I'D LIKE TO THANK MY FRIEND JACKIE BECHER for lighting the fire in me to write this book. She seemed convinced that readers would warm to some of my personal experiences as a woman. When I told my friend and fellow author George Hamilton that I was taking it upon myself to write this book—I mean, really sit down and *write*—he said, "Well, get ready for natural childbirth, without the epidural." He was right! Writing a book is not an easy chore, and even after I finally got into the swing of things, sometimes finding just the right words was an elusive task. It's one of the most difficult of all challenges to express ideas and feelings in writing while hanging on to your own inner voice. I couldn't have managed to do so in a void.

I would like to thank David Vigliano, my literary agent, who responded positively to the idea of a "woman to woman" book from yours truly. With his help, I was fortunate to wind up with a brilliant and insightful publishing team at Weinstein Books, headed by Harvey Weinstein, entrepreneur par excellence. It's been a real joy to work with the combined talents of Judy Hottensen, Kristin Powers, Katie Finch, and Richard Florest. I also thank my longtime manager Steve Sauer, for his unwavering support and guidance; and I so appreciate my friend and colleague, Julie Nathanson, who encouraged me from the outset. Finally, I'm forever grateful to my editor, Bruce Benderson, who over the months helped me stay on track, kept my writer's morale up, and helped me format the book in a cohesive way. He made the whole experience fun.

I'd also like to thank my friends and family, especially Damon and Tahnee, for their patience and understanding throughout this time-consuming process. No words are enough to say thanks to Aurora Jean Mitcham, who is the closest thing to a guardian angel on this earth. And I cannot forget my assistant, Angela, who pulled out all the stops to help and deserves a medal for her daily support.

Photo Credits

Unless otherwise noted, all photos are from the author's collection. Every effort has been made to identify copyright holders; in case of oversight, and on notification to the publisher, corrections will be made in the next edition.

Page ii

One Million Years B.C. (1966): Ronnie Pilgrim © Twentieth Century Fox

Page vi

Maid of California (1956): Courtesy of the San Diego Union Tribune
Raquel Welch, James Welch and Tahnee Welch: © Tim Geaney
Kansas City Bomber (1972): Courtesy of Warner Brothers
Signing autographs w/ Damon: courtesy of David McGough
The Three Musketeers (1973): Terry O'Neill © Twentieth Century Fox
The Wild Party (1975): Courtesy of MGM Studios Inc.
Myra Breckenridge (1970): Terry O'Neill © Twentieth Century Fox

Insert page 5:

Maid of California (1956): Courtesy of the San Diego Union Tribune

Insert page 8:

photo from LIFE magazine: Don Ornitz © Globe Photos Inc.

Insert page 9:

Roustabout: Bud Fraker © Paramount Pictures
Biggest Bundle of Them All (1968): Courtesy of Warner Brothers
100 Rifles (1969): Courtesy of Twentieth Century Fox
One Million Years B.C. (1966): Ronnie Pilgrim © Twentieth Century Fox
Fantastic Voyage (1966): Ted Allan © Twentieth Century Fox

Insert page 10:

Bandolero! (1968): Martin Mills, courtesy of Twentieth Century Fox

Insert page 11:

Raquel & Frank Sinatra: Terry O'Neill © Hulton Archive/Getty Images
100 Rifles (1969): Courtesy of Twentieth Century Fox
Backstage at *Woman Of the Year* (1983): Ron Galella © Wireimage

Insert page 12:

Fantastic Voyage (1966): John Springer © Twentieth Century Fox
Myra Breckenridge (1970): Terry O'Neill © Twentieth Century Fox
The Three Musketeers (1973): Terry O'Neill © Twentieth Century Fox
Signing autographs w/ Damon: courtesy of David McGough
Kansas City Bomber (1972): Courtesy of Warner Brothers
Meeting the Queen: © Bettmann/CORBIS

Insert page 13:

The Wild Party (1975): Courtesy of MGM Studios Inc.
Woman of the Year (1982): © Martha Swope

Insert page 14:

Damon Welch: © Vera Anderson

Permissions

I Wish You Love
English Words by Albert Beach
French Words and Music by Charles Trenet
Copyright © 1946, 1955 by UNIVERSAL MUSIC—
MGB SONGS and EDITIONS SALABERT
Copyright Renewed
All Rights Controlled and Administered in the USA and Canada
by UNIVERSAL MUSIC CORP.
All Rights Reserved. Used by Permission
Reprinted by permission of Hal Leonard Corporation

I'm A Woman
© 1961 Sony/ATV Music Publishing LLC. All rights administered by
Sony/ATV Music Publishing LLC, 8 Music Square West, Nashville, TN 37203